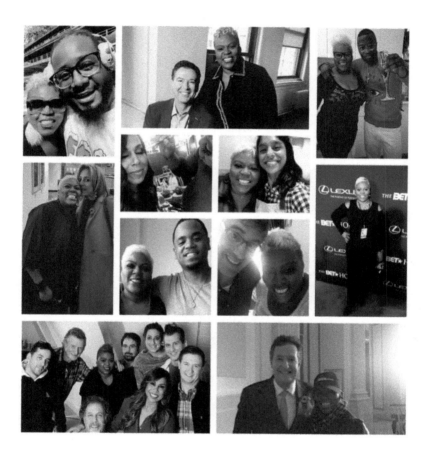

Lipgloss Chronicles

Confessions of a Celebrity Makeup Artist

Mayvis Payne
Foreword by Mo Rocca

To view some of my celebrity clients and portfolio, please visit my website at: www.mayvispayne.com.

Publishing Service By: Pen Legacy®
Cover By: Christian Cuan
Edited By: Candice "Ordered Steps" Johnson
Formatted By: U Can Mark My Word Editorial Services

Library of Congress Cataloging – in- Publication Data has been applied for.

ISBN: 978-1-7366118-9-0

PRINTED IN THE UNITED STATES OF AMERICA.

Dedications

This book is dedicated to two people:

First, to my dearly departed grandmother, Maggie Ora Lee Stanford. In her quiet strength, my grandmother was my very first role model. I've been blessed with her strength; however, I failed to get the *quiet* memo. Although fashion wasn't a concern of hers, my grandmother was adorned with the most regal garment anyone can possess: *inner beauty*. Coupled with her gorgeous smile and pure heart, she was a perfect masterpiece. Thank you for praying over me, Grams, and for the shining example you were to all who knew you.

Secondly, to my biggest fan - my husband, Michael Payne. It was you who encouraged me to pursue my dream of becoming a makeup artist. Likewise, had it not been for your coaxing and cheerleading, this book may not have manifested. Thank you for basically filling every required position I needed for my journey to SUCCESS: driver, web developer, virtual assistant, not-so-willing model, short-order cook, private investigator, coffee runner, bellhop, and financier. *Wait! Do I have to pay you back*? Because of your unwavering love and support, we can now enjoy a life that is cozy, comfortable and complete. Thank you for believing in me.

Lipgloss Chronicles

Confessions of a Celebrity Makeup Artist

Foreword

One of the highest compliments I can be paid by someone I've interviewed is *"You made me feel so comfortable."* I want the person to open up, to tell me who they are, and hopefully to share something they have not told another person outside their family. And if there are tears, even better!

But making someone feel comfortable on camera is never the work of one person. I can be on my game, but if the room is too cold, the light is burning their eyes, or the sound guy digs a little too "in there" to attach the microphone, the person is not going to feel comfortable. A makeup artist is crucial to bringing ease and peace and a general feeling of "this is going to be a good day" to a set, to the guest stars and to, um, the host of a show.

Mayvis Payne brought that peaceful, easy (and joyful) feeling to *"My Grandmother's Ravioli"*, the show I hosted on the Cooking

Mayvis Payne

Channel. On each episode, we traveled into a different senior citizen's kitchen to watch them teach me treasured family recipes while telling me their life story. The cameras were rolling when I actually met each grandparent, a high-stakes moment which made me nervous. We needed to get this right.

On each episode Mayvis was the last person I saw before that on-camera meeting. She would make me up in whatever space was available – the hallway of an apartment building ... the cellar of a house ... inside a van. (Remember, we weren't shooting in a studio.) Not always ideal for her to do her job and yet whatever the circumstance, she turned those twenty minutes into a soothing, meditative, deeply reassuring recess from worry. All those awful things I imagined could go wrong that day fell away and I could focus.

Makeup artistry is so intimate. There's the physical closeness and the trust required. (Okay, I'll keep my eye open if I'm convinced you won't slip and jab my cornea.) But it's more than that. Mayvis was the first person I spent any significant time with on shoot days – and it was her energy I was taking with me in front of the cameras. She knew just what to say – maybe it was some intel on the grandmother I was about to meet, maybe it was something funny that had happened with the crew that morning, maybe it was just saying nothing because that felt right. And then I was ready to fly. She was not unlike the momma bird gently pushing me from the nest.

But Mayvis wasn't just making me up. She also made up my "co-stars", the grandparents. And her magic here was every bit as potent. These were older people who, with few exceptions, *had never been on camera before.* If they weren't confident, the whole show was a bust. And so, when Grandma Kitty in Pittsburgh almost backed out on the morning of her episode's taping, it was Mayvis who made her feel safe. On the opposite end, the ladies of Akron's "Lebron James Grandmothers Fan Club" didn't have cold feet. In fact, I'm not sure there's ever been a more boisterous group. With them Mayvis pulled double duty as makeup artist and chaperone.

Uniformly the show's grandparents loved her because she loved them. Ruth Taube was, at the time of shooting, a 94-year-old lifelong resident of New York's Lower East Side. A tough old bird (and I mean that as the highest praise), Ruth had been widowed during World War II, had once beaten up a man who insulted her daughter, and had spent most of her life teaching sewing skills to immigrants at a settlement house. Ruth was and is glorious – and blunt. In her inimitable way, she had no problem questioning a cameraman or snapping at a crew member that he was off his mark.

But with Mayvis, she surrendered all control. I can still hear Ruth calling "Maaaayvis", asking for a little more blush, a bit more something for the eyes. With her expertise, personality and spirit, Mayvis made Ruth feel special. She made her feel like a star. Mayvis is, as the kids say, a mood. A very, very good one.

I think Ruth was responding to more than Mayvis' excellent technique or her radiant smile – and it is *radiant*. There was a real connection there, a simpatico. Both these women, so far apart in age and different in backgrounds, share something more important. They're both perpetually moving forward, whatever the obstacle. As you'll read in these pages, Mayvis' love for her profession and for people has buoyed her through all kinds of stormy weather.

She has more than a remarkable eye for detail. (I mean, she

Mayvis Payne

is a makeup artist.) She has a clarity of vision. She asks herself the big questions and answers them with courage. She knows in her mind and in her heart that, as she puts it, your gift will make room for you.

I just hope there's room in her chair for me.

Mo Rocca
January 2021
New York City

TABLE OF CONTENTS

Preface

I first met Mayvis in Maryland where we worked together. As I grew to know her prior to becoming a makeup artist, I knew she was going to be a star. She had all the qualities for success: A superstar image, class, charisma, and most importantly, genuineness. I am proud to have been chosen to write this preface to her captivating journey as a celebrity makeup artist. I pray this book inspires you in many areas of your life.

For years, I've been telling Mayvis she needed to share her story/journey with the world. Not only are the experiences recounted in this book entertaining, they're also a helpful guide for others who may be starting in the industry, or seasoned professionals who've been in the professional makeup field for years. Who knows - maybe this will pique someone's interest and encourage them to follow in her footsteps. Perhaps it will inspire them to take a leap of faith and launch the business they've always dreamed of, no matter the field.

Mayvis Payne

Mayvis has mentored several other makeup artists whom I believe are fulfilling their dreams in the makeup industry, thanks to her contributions. The stories shared in this book are captivating and wide ranging, peppered with intriguing memories of life before the brushes. The testimony of how and why she started down the path of her primary profession, and how she shares the ups and downs she experienced while working with clients, celebrities and high-profile individuals are engaging.

For those wondering who she is and why you should read this memoir, let me answer that for you:

Mayvis has over fifteen years of experience in the entertainment industry, with extensive experience in cosmetology and retail beauty, as well as knowledge and insight on how to launch and build a brand. She has her own cosmetics line, has worked with multiple celebrities and influencers in various areas of entertainment: film, stage, television, fashion, and politics. She's also studied and taken classes at home and abroad. Additionally, she is forever reading, researching and studying new methods to hone her craft. Most importantly, Mayvis is someone who makes every client who sits in her chair feel like they've been friends for years.

I'm excited to see what the future holds for Mayvis. I'm equally proud to be the husband of not only a mother, friend, mentor, entrepreneur, boss-babe, and now...author.

Michael Payne

Hidden Passion, Enter Fashion

I'm often asked whether I've always wanted to become a makeup artist.

That one small question has caused me to revisit my past and humble beginnings. Although I have always loved fashion, beauty and frilly things, I didn't consider makeup artistry as a career, per se – it was thrust upon me. While I am now a *Chanel* and *Creed* girl, back in the day, I wore *Jean Naté* and my uncles' *Brut*. (That statement alone ages me).

The answer to the burning question? No. I wanted to be a nurse; however, God had another plan.

I wasn't allowed to wear makeup until late in high school. During this time, I was selected to strut in a high school fashion show, which was produced by a former model. That alone was an utter shock. I was 5'3" (at best), and modeling was never part of my wildest dreams. I wonder why I even entertained it, considering I have always been fearful of the spotlight.

One of the outfits I wore was a pantsuit, sewn by my mother. I will never forget the lavender, double-breasted masterpiece. There was a flap which folded downward, and the underside was a rich cream color. It was literally a showstopper! Mom was a fantastic seamstress, often creating matching outfits for her and me when I was young. She sewed our cheerleader uniforms, crafted wedding dresses and suits...but that funky lavender two-piece was by far my favorite work of art. I can still see the gaped mouths when it was announced my mother had sewn it! Everyone just knew I had purchased it from a fancy department store.

Although I was short and had never modeled before, the producer praised my strut and encouraged me to model more often, and began booking me for modeling gigs at local department stores. I modeled bathing suits, active wear, evening wear, and everything in between. When I hit the stage, my fears automatically vanished. According to my pseudo-agent, I was a natural. For someone who was terrified being out front, I find it fascinating that I achieved that goal. Even to date, I don't like being on stage - unless it's teaching about makeup, of course.

That high school show was my introduction into the world of fashion. I was bitten by the beauty bug, which led to makeup, fashion magazines, couture clothing and the entertainment industry. It was then that I began paying more attention to all things beautiful!

The following year, I was accepted into Barbizon Modeling School. Although I was working and had my own money for tuition, my mother wouldn't allow me to attend. That's another book for another day, but let's just say I showed her - I broke into the industry another way. We relocated from Mississippi to Ohio during my sophomore year of high school and my love for fashion took on another course. Everything was different; the fashion, advanced art and entertainment, even the dialect! Talk about culture shock, but I digress.

During senior year, I had enough credits to take a vocational course, and was accepted into a nursing assistant course. I excelled in the class, and was awarded a full scholarship to the Ohio State University School of Nursing, but another surprise awaited me that summer: I was pregnant. Almost immediately, I decided against going to college and thrust myself into motherhood. Again, another book later.

Many moons later, I enrolled in school, and I now have a couple of college years under my belt. I hope to return to acquire my degree, but in the meantime...

As I reflect on my belief that my steps were ordered to become a makeup artist, I can recall several instances when my past would offer a glimpse of my future.

Each morning while in grade school, I left the house in pigtails; however, the first opportunity I had, I dashed inside the bathroom, took my hair down and slapped on some lip gloss. It was a bold move, but you better believe that before the 3:00 p.m. bell rang, I made sure to get those ponytails back up, and scrubbed my mouth clean. Mom played zero games!

My grade-school teacher and her husband didn't have any biological children, so they adopted me as their Goddaughter. She was stunning and I was drawn to her beauty; she was always well-dressed, complete with a painted face and gorgeous mane of hair which never seemed to be out of place. She regularly took me to the opera, and although I didn't care for the style of singing, I was mesmerized by the elaborate costumes and makeup.

Now Mom constantly bought new outfits for me to wear, which gave me an extra burst of excitement. Dressing up excited me, even if the show bored me to tears. Thinking back, I should've embraced the opportunity to hone my soprano skills, darn it!

Mom and my Godmother tried their best to *culture* me. I was in a drama club, school and church choirs, band and a cheerleader for many years. The latter is likely why my kids accuse me of yelling so much when they were young...*yeah, let's blame it on that*.

I was encouraged to play an instrument, which led to auditioning in various elements: flute, violin, clarinet and piano. I wasn't gifted in any of those areas, so I resolved to enjoy the music, drool over the fashion and leave the playing to the experts.

In addition to my love of music, I had a magazine library out of this world. I've always loved reading as well as flipping through catalogues and album covers, while admiring the latest fashion trends. Back then, everything was so colorful. I still remember the vividness of the *Right On!* Magazine, and I was certain Foster Sylvers was going to propose to me. Although I never mastered the hair-styling thing, my doll-head received the star treatment every week. I filled her hair with foam rollers and used my crayons to draw on makeup. She needed to be meticulously groomed to be in my life.

When I was sixteen, I landed my first job and spent my earnings at the mall. Even then, I was drawn to expensive looking couture clothing. I've always loved wearing heels, and I bought them to match my outfits. I don't know if it's because I'm short, but when I put on a pair of heels, my entire life is made.

Okay that's a bit dramatic, but you get the gist. To this day, my shoe game is on point!

One day I was called to my high school principal's office, where I was advised some of the girls were complaining about my wardrobe. "You dress as if you're going to a nine-to-five," she lamented. "Why don't you wear jeans and sneakers like the other kids?" Jeans and sneakers were never my thing, so I immediately told my mother how insulted I was. Well... I can't print Mom's conversation with the principal, but she never spoke to me again.

I've always had an eye for fashion. It still baffles me, though that I cannot draw or paint (outside of faces), but I somehow manage to put things nicely together. Although I didn't immediately pursue a career in fashion, I was often complimented about my clothing and home decor. Having always been drawn to unique clothing and style, if someone else had it - I didn't want it.

This tradition continued throughout my life, even as I conducted several "dress rehearsals" to prep my daughter for school dances and proms. I played music, poured sparkling cider and applied her makeup as if I were creating a masterpiece. It was a production, I tell you! She looked like I'd completely lost it, but I was having so much fun.

What in the world is going on, my daughter wondered? *Why is Mom being so extra?*

Now we know...passion!

Many years later, following a divorce, my two children and I moved to Maryland, where I accepted a job that would be a fresh start for me and also a great place to introduce my children to the advancement of the African American culture. As a quality control inspector, I worked extremely close with the engineering department, located in a separate building. Oftentimes while visiting that location, I casually exchanged greetings with a handsome, well-dressed man, which usually went no further than *hello*. After three and a half years of quick greetings, one day he finally struck up a conversation with me and eventually we became really good friends.

One year later, my position was eliminated. That's such a cute term...actually, I was rifted. Six months afterwards, my *greeter* and I began dating. We dated a year before we married and twenty years later, he's still my biggest cheerleader. I am a successful makeup artist today because my husband appreciated my passion for beauty and pushed me to pursue it as a career.

After losing my job, I re-entered corporate America as a sales and marketing assistant in Washington D.C., then as an administrative assistant for the Energy Consulting Group at the prestigious Deloitte. My husband and I commuted by train, and on numerous occasions, I received compliments from other women about my makeup. After more than four years of hearing "Your makeup is beautiful," a light bulb went off:

Perhaps I should study makeup artistry.

I had a great job, with fantastic pay and benefits, and my husband had a fruitful career; however, I felt there was something more I should be doing.

Besides knowing that MAC makeup was all the craze, I didn't know much about makeup or how to pursue a career in it. Until this time, I don't think I even considered how makeup artists played such a crucial role in the industry. Eventually, I researched makeup schools in the area, but what I found only frustrated me. Every school I found only allowed students to study makeup along with another skill, like hair or nails. I wasn't interested in learning either of those, so I shunned the idea of enrolling.

Speaking of being shunned:

Soon after I ditched the idea of furthering my education, perfect timing allowed me to bump into a popular celebrity makeup artist at an event I attended out of town. When I asked if she was familiar with any good schools, she shunned me. (You'll hear more about her in a later chapter). Anyway, her reaction fueled my fire.

I began researching again.

Honestly, I'm not certain whether I expected my pursuit to lead to anything, but the more I researched, the more excited I became. I settled on a school in Annapolis, Maryland - Chesapeake School of Esthetics and Makeup Artistry. My plan was to take the makeup artistry course first, then return to study esthetics. That was MY plan; God had something else for me.

In 2003, I made the sacrifice to attend the summer courses. We owned one vehicle at the time, and I had to get off work early two days each week to drive from D.C. to Annapolis. My husband rode the train, then either hailed a taxi or walked home to tend to our teenage children. Shout out to my husband for that feat alone!

As for the class, there was a seven-to-one student-teacher ratio. The first night of class, I was a bundle of nerves and excitement. Until that day, I thought I had a general understanding of makeup. I knew NOTHING…except I wasn't going to last. Thank God I was wrong.

The inaugural class was one of the best learning experiences I've ever had. The instructor was gorgeous, highly knowledgeable, and approachable. Likewise, she was patient, and knew how to extract talent from her students. One evening as we were preparing to leave, my instructor called out, "Mayvis just looks like a makeup artist!" That single statement gave me the boost of confidence that I needed.

Mayvis Payne

We were encouraged to attend beauty conferences and start considering which area of work to pursue. To help with that, our instructor maintained an updated list of job openings, but for some odd reason, I never followed up on any leads. I think I was still unconvinced that I really wanted a career. I did attend the beauty shows, though. After the first show in Florida, I instantly realized I wanted to earn a living doing makeup. Following graduation, I had no idea how to break into the industry; however, the first thing I did was have business cards printed. My first cards were colorful, and included a photo of me with bright blue eyeshadow. Thinking how awful that card must've appeared to potential clients, I shudder…but I passed them out with pride. I had no shame - no job board, supermarket, or gym was safe.

No place was off limits; I passed those hideous cards out like M&Ms!

Artist Tip

- **Be sure to maintain an arsenal of professional materials showcasing your brand and craft, i.e., website business cards portfolio etc.**
- **Even when you're clueless, go hard for your business. Know that your steps are already ordered, and you can achieve your goals.**

Retail, Re-Tell

B y now, MAC was the only cosmetics brand I used. One day, I decided to shop at the Georgetown location where a stunning, young African American lady assisted me with my purchases. When I arrived home, I discovered she placed an extra item of significant value in my bag, but failed to charge me for it. I double-checked my receipt to make sure I hadn't been charged, then called the store to inform her what happened, and that I'd be returning.

"Oh wow," she exclaimed, "no one has ever been so honest."

I drove back to Georgetown (a hike from my home), and as I prepared to leave, something came over me.

"Are you guys hiring?" I asked.

"As a matter of fact, we are."

She informed me she was the store manager, and that many

locations – including the one I was in, had openings. I completed the application and returned home, not really expecting to hear back.

Now I thoroughly enjoyed working as an administrative assistant and made a good salary, so I wasn't aggressively seeking work in makeup artistry. But one day while in the office, I received a call from a MAC recruiter, requesting an interview. What?! I was excited and nervous as I arrived at the swanky hotel for the extensive interview, where the meeting was long, but it went okay.

I left the hotel, relieved it was over. With zero retail experience and extraordinarily minimal makeup experience outside of school, I just knew I'd never get a callback. A week later…I was called in for a second interview. This time, my skills would be assessed, and I needed my own model.

I recruited a friend from work as my model, and headed to the Virginia pro store for the demonstration. I was a complete bundle of nerves, so I was relieved when the interviewer was too busy to hover over me. I worked until I felt confident the makeup application was a good representation of my skills, then called for the rep. She quietly evaluated my work, saying I'd done a good job. That's when she turned to my model.

"How do you think she did?" she asked.

"She's done better," my *friend* replied.

I was flabbergasted, shocked and mad all at the same time. Game over…the opportunity I hoped for was gone.

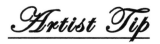

Artist Tip

- **Beware of friends disguised as haters. More examples to follow.**

- **Make sure to be selective and vigilant with whom you share your dreams/goals/vision.**

One day as I sat at my desk, the phone rang. Imagine my surprise to hear MAC's regional leader on the other end. *Thanks, but no thanks*, I braced myself to hear. But the shock was on me: I was offered a position, and training would begin the following week.

The training was two weeks - three days the first week, two the next.

"I'm required to put my request in at least two weeks in advance," I informed her. "I'm not sure I can do it."

"Well if you want to work for us, that's what you're going to have to do."

I don't know how I talked my supervisor into it, but my leave was approved.

I was on my way to becoming a coveted makeup artist for the hottest brand in the world!

Reflecting on my first day of training, I can see the hand of God orchestrating the favor that was extended to me. That day, the trainer went around the room, asking everyone to share their experience with the recruiting process. There were 20 of us; each one recounted how it took anywhere from three to eight interviews before finally getting hired. They gasped in awe when I shared I only interviewed once and was hired. The funny thing is, I was the oldest person in the room - even older than the trainer.

Oh yeah, this was God's doing!

I was hired to work the counter of a brand-new store. As a result, I had to learn the products, help to build the counter, navigate through store protocol, and identify personnel…all while learning about the retail industry.

What have I gotten myself into?

The thought crossed my mind, but I have never been a quitter.

When the store opening arrived, all the company's executives were in house to assist and critique our skills. I invited every woman I knew to drop in for a makeover. Although I was green and not yet a great artist, I had mad confidence, as well as basic knowledge of makeup application. When I tell you my church family showed up on my behalf; every time I glanced up, another one was in the never-ending line for a makeover. Whenever the regional team lead approached them, my supporters quipped, "I'm waiting for Mayvis."

At the end of the day, guess who had the most sales?

It felt so good to have the regional leader pull me aside to congratulate me. What a feeling!

When I joined the beauty team, my aspiration was to become a trainer, but as I progressed, those goals evaporated. I became painfully aware of retail quotas, corporate politics and the intense pressure to sell more. I wanted no parts of it - the mandate to sell, sell, sell, snuffed the fun out. Talent was secondary to performance, and my goals were only important to me; retail companies have their own goals to meet.

Some of the things I saw and heard left an indelible impact upon me as an aspiring artist. That doesn't make the company, nor its structure a bad thing - that's just the nature of the beast and I decided it would not work for me. I have nothing but great respect for my retail experiences, because they're partly responsible for the success I enjoy today. I entered the beauty business just five months after completing makeup school. It's a fast-paced assignment, and I learned a wealth of information and tricks of the trade. The thing I enjoyed most though, was seeing how a simple makeover could shift a woman's outlook. While in my chair, I've literally had women spill their deepest secrets, then burst into tears when I hand them a mirror to see their transformation.

Women confided in me that their spouses called them ugly, unattractive, and unworthy. I've encountered significant others who wouldn't allow their women to wear makeup.

Which reminds me of a young lady I made over who was in her early 20s. She purchased two hundred dollars' worth of cosmetics I used on her. The next morning as I opened the store, a handsome young gentleman approached me, saying he had a return.

The bag he handed over to me was the purchase the young lady from the previous day made.

Every.single.item.returned.

When he left, I shook my head, pondering how a woman so young was already being controlled by a boyfriend who hadn't even committed to being her husband! I shouldn't have been shocked – she'd already confessed how he didn't want her wearing makeup, which I'd hear often throughout the years.

My response?

"But how do YOU feel when you wear makeup?"

To me, that's what matters. Makeup isn't for everybody, however if a little lip gloss or mascara makes you feel good - go for it!

One of the greatest lessons I've learned in my journey is

people don't necessarily buy into your products - they buy into you. She likely had no intention of making such a vast purchase, but the experience she encountered encouraged her to do so.

More on this later.

Although I wasn't the best artist, I was always one of the top sellers at the various locations I worked during my tenure. I believe that people trusted I wasn't manipulating them to make unnecessary purchases, but instead offering what they needed (whether it was cosmetics or a listening ear).

In spite of the numbers-obsessed retail industry, with its pressure to increase revenue, I believe in honesty and integrity. Gaining the confidence and trust of a client/customer means having their support for life. Every week, falling short of sales goals stressed many of my colleagues. Because I was usually ahead of my goals, I handed over some of my sales for them to ring up as their own. I recall doing a makeover one time, when I overheard my coworkers talking.

Colleague 1: "Mayvis always makes her goal."

Colleague 2: "Yes, but have you seen her customer service? She's the best!"

They weren't aware I heard them; however, I snagged the opportunity to coach them a bit. After the customer left, I broached the subject of sales and customer service with my colleagues. The first colleague often shunned customers whom she considered to be non-spenders, or didn't *look the part*.

"Do you know why you guys struggle with making your goals?" I asked. "First of all, you're famous for assuming certain customers are cheap. Maybe they don't plan to purchase anything today, but if you give them excellent customer service, they may change their mind.

"Or maybe they don't have the money to buy what they want today," I went on, "but if you treat them like queens anyway, they'll come back to spend their money with you."

As the *mother* of most of the counters I worked, I often found myself dropping knowledge. Sometimes it fell on deaf ears, sometimes they listened. In any event, I'm grateful for my experiences as a retail artist. I was taught invaluable lessons which also prepared me for the ruthless entertainment industry.

Artist Tip

- **Life lessons are everywhere - pay attention.**

I was hired as a part time artist, so I kept my full-time job. Being a part-timer, I worked two to three days during the week, and every Saturday (the busiest retail day), and sometimes Sunday, too. In addition to the strict weekend rule, the company also had a *not-one-minute* late policy. Now I'm a stickler for time, so that wasn't a challenge, but navigating through D.C./Maryland traffic to clock in on time was excruciating. Thankfully, I never clocked in late; not once! (Back in those days, companies actually used time clocks, so your time was accurately documented. Talk about old school).

During this time, my husband and I shared a car. When I was in school, we drove to D.C. to secure street parking on class days. As if that wasn't stressful enough, I had to set my alarm on my work computer to remind me to put money in the parking meter every two hours to avoid getting a ticket, because those meter maids are extremely prompt and thorough! On top of all of this, I had to get off work early to get to class on time. Man, I'm so grateful for angels shielding me from state troopers, because when I tell you I hit at least ninety miles per hour trying to get there on time, please believe it!

On my retail workdays, I left my full-time job early, took the train to my husband's job downtown, and drove the car back to Maryland. It was such a struggle! I would like to pause to salute my husband Mike, my biggest supporter. Were it not for him believing in my vision, none of this would have worked.

I absolutely loved my day job, and worked my butt off on a daily basis. It is difficult to navigate corporate politics and creativity, both at the same time, but I juggled so effortlessly, that it looked easy. I supported heavy-hitting partners and directors; however, working with the Energy Group was simultaneously rewarding and challenging. *Well, most of the time it was rewarding.*

Imagine working 8 a.m. to 5 p.m., then working another job from 6 p.m. to 10 p.m. I was oftentimes drained. Even though my shift ended at 10 p.m., we had to completely clean the counters before leaving for the night. Most nights, I didn't get out until after 11 p.m., then drove home to my family, who were in bed by then. I managed to get a few hours of sleep, only to start all over again the next day.

Cosmetics was the busiest of all the departments, and no other counter could leave until we were finished. Often, customers lingered until the very last minute, before we could even begin shutting down. The other counters glared and cursed us out as we thoroughly cleaned, ticked they had to wait for us. I can still hear our department manager screaming at the top of her lungs, "MAC, hurry up!"

By the way, that manager later became one of our best customers and eventually stopped giving us so much grief.

…but it took a minute.

I'd been working with the company for about six months when my husband suggested I should drop my day job and work exclusively in retail beauty. I protested, reminding him we were saving for a house, had one car and I was making great money. I'll never forget his response:

"If you're not happy, what good is it?" he questioned. "I've watched you being dog tired when you get off work at your full-time job, but on days when you're scheduled to do makeup, you light up and suddenly have a burst of energy."

When I shared my husband's sentiments with my best friend, she co-signed his suggestion. "God doesn't need your full-time job to give you a house," she said.

I pondered their advice, but continued working. In my heart, I knew they were right, but I concluded that I needed the job to finance my dream.

By now I didn't enjoy my day job as much as I once had. I adored the people, and loved the money, but I felt unappreciated, bored and empty. Our close friends badgered me about being a full-time makeup artist, and my response was always a resounding NO. I understood retail is about selling. If you don't sell, you don't eat. That was my crutch for hanging on to my full-time job, which meant working with a partner who'd become difficult to deal with.

Around this time, my husband, I, and four of our friends attended a jazz festival where one of my favorite artists was singing. We were having an incredible time, when she suddenly stopped singing.

Mayvis Payne

"You know what? Sometimes you just have to step out on faith," she said, going on to share how she quit her job to pursue her career. She mentioned her opportunities didn't come until after she stretched her faith and quit her job. All our friends turned and stared at me. I smiled, but cringed inside.

The next morning as the pastor delivered the sermon in church, he proclaimed, "Sometimes you have to step out on faith."

I hear you, God.

When we arrived home, I advised my hubby I received confirmation to quit my full-time job and submitted my resignation the next day. I gave two weeks' notice; however, they requested I stay to train my replacement. I consented, remaining longer than anticipated. All of my superiors were aware of my leaving, and the *difficult one* sent me an email.

HIM: Hi, Mayvis. I heard that you're leaving for another opportunity. Congratulations! Does this new opportunity have anything to do with the makeup classes you were taking?

ME: Thank you for the well wishes. I'm leaving because of you.

(Blunt honesty is my strong suit.)

I'm certain he wasn't expecting that response; I wished I could've seen his face when he read it. He was accustomed to being the rude one; never on the receiving end.

I finished training the new assistant, collected my severance package, and vacationed in Cancun for nine days

34

with Mike. While away, I picked up a greeting card and mailed it to my estranged former boss. I scribbled on the inside of the blank card: **Thank You, Mayvis Payne.**

Sidebar: About a year later, we bumped into each other in a bookstore and engaged in a pleasant conversation. As he introduced me to his wife and children, he shared how proud he was of me, that I had pursued my dream.

See, afterwards I realized that man was a pawn in my life's game of chess. No bad feelings were warranted; he was instrumental in pushing me towards destiny.

One of my other partners and I had a great working relationship, and his wife called and stopped in to see me from time to time, bringing gifts with her. I had often shared my dream of becoming a makeup artist with that partner. Although I had no intentions of working with celebrities at the time, I blurted, "You'll see my name in lights one day," as I exited.

A couple of weeks after I resigned, I was booked to do makeup for an *X-Men 3* press junket. The studio was a couple of blocks from my old job, so when I finished with the *X-Men cast*, I stopped by to say hello. I arrived with a fancy new hairdo, heavy makeup and trendy attire, prompting my favorite partner to ask what I was up to. When I told him I just finished making up the *X Men* cast, he gasped.

"Damn, I knew you would do big things, but I didn't know it would be so soon!" he exclaimed.

"Told you so," I laughed.

As it turned out, my best friend was right. God didn't need a job where I was miserable to bless me with a house. The following spring, after I'd been in the beauty business for a year, we moved into our very first home, perched in a nice

Mayvis Payne

Maryland suburb.

I was a part-time retail artist and loved my job, but it felt like a full-time position. Shortly after being hired, it was announced that our manager was leaving, and I was asked if I'd like to fill the position. "Thanks, but no thanks," I replied. I didn't want to do this full-time. I'd seen how things were done (and not done), ultimately deciding I wanted no parts of management. I was sad to see my manager leave, though. She was fun, personable, fair, and an incredible artist!

One day after opening the store, I was the only employee on the floor for a couple of hours.

In walked the manager, with a bare face.

"Good morning," she chirped. "I want you to do my makeup."

If that wasn't nerve-wrecking enough, she added, "I want a smokey eye."

What?

Smokey eyes were a challenge for me. I'd never applied them before, and didn't want to now. "I'm not good with smokey eyes," I confessed.

"I know - that's why you're going to practice on me."

My hands trembled as I began her application. She didn't say a word while I worked, but she politely critiqued me when I was finished. I didn't do as badly as I had thought (thank God), and her advice gave me the confidence I needed. The smokey eye became one of my most requested applications.

Shout out to wonderful retail beauty managers.

Moments like these helped shape my career. I made tons of mistakes as a retail artist, but those stumbling blocks became my stepping stones to success. I still cringe seeing photos of

36

some of my early applications, but I also see the growth. I'm forever grateful to my former colleagues, managers and customers for allowing me the room to bloom and not holding my errors against me. Some of my former colleagues tell me customers still come in, asking about me. That within itself is a testament to the type of excellent service I strived to offer.

Many customers came in ready to make purchases worth hundreds; however, if I wasn't working, they left and didn't come back until I was there. Those customers kept my sales goals in the positive; it was impossible not to forge relationships with them. They trusted me, and often invited me to gatherings, weddings, church, etc.

One such customer was a pastor's wife. She didn't even wear makeup, but spent hundreds of dollars with me each time she came in. Later, she told me she gifted the makeup and brushes to the women at her church. I loved Mrs. Young!

Working the counter also taught me how to deal with difficult, hesitant or aloof customers.

For example:

A woman wandered into the store, searching for a good skincare and makeup regimen. Upon listening to her concerns, I walked with her around the counter, suggesting products and offered a demonstration. She wasn't interested in having her makeup done, and didn't really seem to be receptive of my recommendations. I mean, talk about poker face! I couldn't read her.

Once I finished my spill, the woman said, "Okay - I'll take everything."

I remained cool, but my mouth was probably wide open.

"Yes ma'am, let me bag everything for you," I replied,

totaling the purchase in my head. I was excited - my goal was met for the week! As I tallied the items, I waited for her to decline some of them, but she didn't. The transaction totaled a few hundred dollars, and she requested a business card. I made a practice of keeping both my company issued card and personal card on hand, so I handed over both. Turns out the woman was a producer for a major network, and was going to refer me to do makeup for their shows.

Knock me over with a mascara wand!

I was dumbfounded. This goes back to my mantra - always extend excellent customer service and be nice to everyone, because you never know whom you're servicing. This lady was dressed down in casual attire, complete with a baseball cap and totally unassuming. She did exactly what she said she would, and to date, we're still friends – a rarity in this business.

Throughout my years as a contractor with the network, she often stopped by the makeup room to chat and check on me. In addition, she has attended a few of my makeup classes and has purchased some of my products. I'll never forget her. Undoubtedly, she's responsible for introducing me to the world of television makeup artistry, and I'm forever grateful.

Artist Tip

- **Despise not small beginnings, and treat everyone with kindness. You never know where it will lead.**

I was completely green as a freelance artist, but my name was gaining traction, so I was quickly integrated into the game. During this time, a man representing himself as an agent for makeup artists called me about joining his agency. Without ever meeting me, he emailed an agreement letter, and began booking me for projects. He called often, claiming to have a huge celebrity or high-profile client for me, but it always fell through. Later, I discovered this back and forth was part of his shady routine.

For the next few months, the "agent" occasionally booked several gigs for me, mostly with television. I looked up to him because he was doing his thing in the industry. We spoke almost daily, sometimes several times a day. After a while, he invited me to a meet-and-greet with other makeup artists working for him as well. I was booked one to two days a week; the money was so good, I left part-time retail (freelancing only when I was available) and joined his agency. This helped me focus on pursuing a career as an industry artist, while keeping my foot in the door with a cosmetics brand, working when it was convenient to my schedule.

After working with the agency for seven months, my gigs and conversations with the agent started making me uneasy. Some things just didn't add up. On one occasion, he booked me to style a lead anchor for a major network in New York. She absolutely loved her makeup, and mentioned that she'd been invited to the White House the next day. When she asked if I'd do her makeup for the event, I was ecstatic! I agreed, handing her the agency business card, which only included the agent's contact information.

At her request, I gave her my name and promptly called the

agent to advise him I'd been booked. His demeanor was odd, but he played it off by saying it was a great opportunity and it was good to be personally requested by this client. Now in our written agreement, artists could not accept work or contact clients, so I followed protocol and advised the client to contact the agent for approval. The look on her face said she didn't like that rule, either.

I was so green.

The next day, the agent was booked for a gig and asked if I could relieve him for about two hours. Guess whose makeup he left to go do? The client who requested ME. I never said another word about it; however, I never heard from that particular client again.

While it was well within the agent's right to prohibit freelancers from pursuing his clients, I often wondered why he poached her. How many other clients had requested me? What did he say when they asked? This was my introduction to the unscrupulous antics of the industry, and there would be many more. I paid closer attention to what he said, how he responded, and more importantly, how I conducted business with him going forward.

Following this incident, I was booked for a huge client for two days. After undergoing a strict background check, I arrived at the trailer. This was my very first time working in a trailer, but it wouldn't be the last.

Sidebar: Trailers are usually too cold or too hot – nothing in between...

For this job, I was making over television reporters. Working in trailers is vastly different from the posh comforts of the green room, but I was on cloud nine. I wouldn't have cared if I was slinging my brushes in a closet! A few hours later, a young woman wandered in and introduced herself to me. She was incredibly young - much younger than me, she grew up in the industry, and had a wealth of experience, knowledge and insight. As we shared our experiences with each other, she said something which took me aback, but has remained with me throughout my professional career. Even though I was flabbergasted at the time, many years later, I would eventually agree:

"In this industry, everybody lies."

Her observation struck me like an open-handed slap to the face. Had I heard her correctly? Did she mean *everyone*? The definitive way it poured from her lips assured me she meant it. Years later, I echoed the same sentiment. Although I've worked with some honest and integral people, I approach every situation with caution, remembering her words: "In.this.industry.everybody.lies."

Early in my career, I heard about an opportunity to do makeup for a fashion show. I contacted the coordinator and was scheduled to complete a makeup demonstration and interview. The next day, I received the call that I was hired, and more information would be forthcoming. A stipend of one hundred dollars was offered - each artist was assigned ten faces. Prior to the event, I was contacted by the coordinator to inform me the terms had changed. In lieu of payment, I would receive "exposure."

Exposure: *Consider this a profane term.*

Ten thousand people were anticipated to be in attendance at the event, including a high-profile rapper who was performing. The host was a celebrity designer, and other local designers would be featured. I may have been green, but I was neither stupid, nor desperate, therefore I declined the gig with peace. A few minutes after hanging up, I received a call from the celebrity designer. The conversation went something like this:

"Hey, Mayvis! I hear you're not going to participate in my show?"

"That's correct," I confirmed.

"Why not?" disappointment coated his voice.

"Because I was initially told that I would be paid, but now I'm not." I waited a few beats, almost hearing the wheels turning in his head.

"We're going to pay you," he finally said. "Cash - after the show."

Now my wheels spun. "How much, and for how many models?"

"One hundred and fifty dollars," he said quickly, as if I would change my mind before he gave me a number. "How many models do you want to do?"

"Five to six. That's it," I sang with ease, confidence swelling.

"Cool. See you then."

I was impressed that he called me directly, and even more so that I negotiated my own terms. This was great for my résumé, and the experience would be invaluable.

The day of the show arrived, and my hubby dropped me off at the venue. Gazing at the huge venue, I grew nervous. I located the makeup room where a slew of models raced around, and set up my station. There were eight artists to what seemed like one hundred models.

I'm only doing five or six models, I thought as I observed the chaos.

When I started my faces, I noticed the work of the other artists. Man, they were good! Insecurity deflated my spirit; I was in way over my head, I thought. Before I could bolt out of there, one of the designers came over to introduce himself to me. I played it cool when he lamented how much he loved my work and wanted to hire me for an upcoming show, but inside I screamed. Me? Did he not see the other artists' masterpieces?

A couple of the other artists overheard our conversation, and asked if he needed more artists. When he said no, I immediately felt the daggers their scowls shot at me. I remained focused and finished my models, then packed my things along with a few other artists whom I'd become friendly with, and went to watch the show.

My first red flag was the 150 to 200 people in the audience. *What happened to the thousands of people they were expecting*?

Maybe the audience was out front waiting to get in, or running late. Speaking of running late - so was the show.

It was over an hour behind schedule, and the headliner was nowhere in sight. When he eventually arrived, the venue was barely half-full. Nevertheless, I was excited because this was my first gig featuring a celebrity entertainer. I was geeked!

...but my excitement was short lived.

When the show concluded, I mentioned to my colleague that I was going to collect my pay. That's when I learned none of the other makeup artists were getting paid anything other than that wonderful amount of exposure. That taught me to keep my mouth shut.

I shrugged off the awkwardness between the artist and me, and went to collect my money. I approached the designer, asking for my pay so I could leave. Perturbed, he sneered and walked off. I wasn't about to be ignored, so I followed behind him, again requesting my money.

He whirled around, fire spitting from his eyes. "Look here sweetheart, I'm busy. Catch up with me later."

"I want my money," I demanded. "I've done what I agreed to do, now I want to get paid."

I was fuming. How dare he play with my money *and* call me sweetheart?

He motioned to two burly dudes (I'm guessing his bodyguards) who rushed over to us. "Handle her," he commanded, and literally ran off.

"Do we have a problem?" One of his brutes asked, hovering over me like the mob.

"My problem is I want my money," I spat before taking off in pursuit of the designer. I yanked my phone out, and called my husband in hysterics. When he answered I hollered, "Stand by the phone, because I might be going to jail tonight!"

Hubby admonished me to settle down and explain what happened. I hurriedly explained the situation and that I'd call him back, as the designer rushed into the room where the models, designers, handlers and everyone involved in the production were gathered.

I tapped him on the shoulder. "I want my money."

Ignoring me again, he turned to one of his assistants. "Would you please handle her?"

"You can do this later," she told me. "Don't be unprofessional."

That's when I saw red. "I don't even know you, and this ain't your concern," I screamed. Then it was the designer's turn to feel my wrath, and I went ballistic on that dude. I have zero recollection of exactly what I said, but I do know I let loose. I was all the way out there now, and there was no turning back.

A hush quieted the entire room as he stood there looking pitiful while I wreaked havoc. A beautiful young lady approached me with caution in the middle of my tirade. "I'm one of the promoters," her calm tone was a complete contrast to my anger. "Come with me and I'll give you your money." Then she turned to the designer. "I'll deal with you later."

She escorted me to the ATM in the downstairs lobby in silence, as I marched behind her, fuming.

"How much did he promise you?" She asked with her back to me as she inserted a card into the machine.

"One hundred and fifty dollars." Saying it out loud made it seem so small, but the principle overrode the amount.

To my relief, she handed me money with a little extra. I asked her name and thanked her, then returned to the same room to gather my belongings and left. I didn't care if the money had to be printed right then and there; somebody was going to cough it up.

Let this be a lesson to aspiring makeup artists: get the agreement in writing. Don't come out of character like I did. Reflecting back, I probably could have handled the situation better; however, had I not been persistent, I may never have gotten my money.

Sadly, I've heard so many similar stories of artists being duped. This is why the state of New York passed the *Freelancing Isn't Free Act*. See, there were so many production companies stiffing artists on their wages, it was pathetic. How I wish I could tell you this was my only occasion of having to track down my money, but unfortunately, it isn't.

Throughout my career, I kept hearing my colleague's sentiment ringing out... In this industry, everybody lies. *She*

Mayvis Payne

wasn't lying…

In the early stages of my cosmetic brand, a producer said she was so in love with my glosses, she wanted to send some to Oprah, whom she claimed to have worked with. I put together a nice gift box containing my top sellers, along with my business cards and a thank-you note.

When she received my presentation, she said the packaging needed to be redone. I went out and purchased luxury packaging, designer labels and custom-made cards. When I sent her a photo of the new packaging, she said it was perfect and that she'd return the glosses so I could include them. Not only did she *not* return the glosses, she stopped taking my calls – even though she was posting selfies wearing my glosses all over social media!

…and there's more.

Shortly after I relocated to New York, I received a call to do a major celebrity's makeup for an early morning television appearance. I completed the work - but it took months to get paid. As a last resort, I researched my way to the person at the helm of the organization, and sent him a private message via Facebook. Within a week, I had my check. Now this wasn't a gig I solicited - they sought me…but I still had to jump through hoops to get paid.

Getting stiffed one time too many times taught me not to operate without a contract. Child, I won't even do a prom makeover without the terms spelled out. It's best to document the terms in writing, and carefully review the paperwork prior to accepting the assignment. There are a lot of unscrupulous people in this industry. My advice is to beware and don't become one of them.

Artist Tip

- **Be sure to get written agreements/contracts. Carefully read and reread. If there are questions, ask for clarification.**

My introduction to film was thrust upon me and was less dramatic. Remember the young lady who had cautioned me about the industry? She was working on a project, and when it was time to select the makeup artist, she recommended me.

The project was an indie film in Washington, D.C., slated to shoot for ten to fifteen days. The salary was more than I made since becoming an artist, so I was stoked. The film - *Jazz in the Diamond District*, told the story of young Jazz, who was engulfed by the Go-Go music scene in D.C. I didn't know much about the Go-Go music nor the film industry, but I jumped in with both feet. I was immediately hooked by Go-Go myself, and it is one of my favorite genres of music. It's a whole vibe. Shout-out to D.C.!

During the long hours of filming, I met some incredible people, including well-known actors Clifton Powell and Wood Harris. They were complete gentlemen, down-to-earth and extremely easy to work with. My first film was an absolute delight. Although I went for days without seeing my husband, the adrenaline I had onset was intoxicating. After making up the actors and actresses, there was plenty of downtime. Even though I'd be exhausted, I stayed ready to spring to action when called on set. Throughout my career, I've adopted the mantra to always stay ready. I never want the talent, producer or coordinator searching for me when a touch-up is needed.

Mayvis Payne

Once, I was hired by a production company from another state who obtained my résumé. I was asked to bring along an assistant, so I reached out to another artist whom I'd recently worked with on another gig.

She kept disappearing from set, and when she stuck around, her head was buried in her phone, browsing social media. The producer seemed unaware of it, so I let it slide. He thanked me after wrapping; however, I didn't get the warm and fuzzies, so I chalked it up as a closed contact.

The next day, I received an email from the producer, expressing how much he loved my talent and, wait for it…my *professionalism*. He complimented me for being readily available and attentive, then welcomed any opportunity to have me on set again. He never mentioned the assistant, and never emailed her. (I asked her.) Each time he returned to the area, he booked me but never requested an assistant again.

Artist Tip

- **It's unprofessional to step away for personal, non-urgent phone calls, take a smoke break or anything else that makes you unavailable or MIA during filming. If a bathroom break is a must, advise the director or producer and immediately return afterwards.**

After a few years, I was a lot clearer about the industry. And I no longer had an "agent."

Sidebar: The split from the agent came to a disastrous end. He wrote me a scathing letter, said he'd make sure I never got hired again because he was well-connected. Not only did I

48

work consistently in spite of his attempted curse, one of his clients hired me to replace him, after abruptly terminating his contract. A few years later, he would be sued by two of the other artists he had introduced me to at his meet-and-greet.

Karma, much?

That situation confirmed what I already knew: My fate's in nobody's hands except God's. Although the industry is big - He is bigger!

During this time, I continued freelancing in retail, consistently meeting new customers and clients. Makeup artists should always understand the difference between clients and customers and act accordingly. There's no cookie-cutter blueprint, so do your research and carve out a niche that works for *your* business.

While working the counter one day, I assisted a woman who requested makeup for an on-camera appearance. After chatting with her and assisting with her purchase, she asked if I was available to apply her makeup for the appearance. That single encounter led to me becoming the go-to makeup artist for the production company who produced the piece. Before long, I was doing makeup for university commercials, professional sporting teams, celebrity athletes, and PSA's.

The production company shared my contact information with another company, where I began working projects with heavy hitters. Some of the gigs included visiting celebrity homes, which sometimes resulted in having dinner with them, accompanying them on outings and/or being introduced to their families.

During several projects, I've had the opportunity to connect and form relationships with the famous and their circles. Now on a few occasions, I discovered I didn't really like the person after working with them. Television personalities can be strikingly different people up close. I made up my mind early on that I was hired to do a job - my personal affinity didn't matter. As far as they knew, they were my favorite person to work with. That's the attitude I've adopted, which remains to this day.

I remember a time when I was hired to groom a celebrity, whom I was excited to work with. The client was rude, unprofessional and unpolished; the mere thought of giving them touch ups was repulsing. As I sat nearby, I constantly reminded myself I was getting paid (handsomely, I might add) to ease my irritation. I had to suck it up and deal with it, but I soldiered through, making a mental note never to work with them again, if at all possible.

One thing I learned early in my career has tremendously helped me navigate this fickle industry: celebrities are human. They're flawed, have bad days and sometimes, just want to be a *normal* person. Now, I know I can't allow an isolated incident to distort my view of the person. I don't do everything right all the time, and shouldn't expect anyone else to, either. That being said, I have to protect my peace, therefore if I need to decline an offer, I will. In my early years, I did not have this option; now I do.

I'm not star struck, which has made celebrities comfortable around me. They see so much counterfeit in their world, it's refreshing to have genuine people around. Several of them have said I put them completely at ease, so they can relax. When I was a newbie, there was a celebrity client whose wife invited me to dinner a couple of weeks after his assignment with me - just she and I. We met at a nice restaurant, and enjoyed dinner and simply shooting the breeze. I've since lost contact with her, but we met often to hang out. She was totally out of my league: designer shoes, clothes, posh handbags, famous friends, expensive perfumes; however, she was comfortable enough with regular-old me to chill. I never mentioned her famous husband or discussed anything personal, and we shared a nice bond. I realized I offered a safe place for her and I was satisfied with it. It's moments like these that remain with you, more than anything else.

Many years (and assignments) later, I was hired for a television pilot. It was a two-day gig, and the set was filled with the production crew, and network executives. Most of the time, I'm the only female in the room; however, this time, one of the executives was a beautiful young woman. Girl power! We never interacted with one another, but on the last day, she commented how she liked my hair. I thanked her, production wrapped, and I left. A week later, she sent an email asking if I could recommend a good hair stylist. I gave her my recommendation, she thanked me, and life continued. Six months later, I received a call from a producer, who was seeking an artist for an upcoming shoot. She said I came highly recommended by someone. Do you know who that person was? You guessed it: the executive from the pilot.

Later, the executive said she was impressed by how I carried out my duties and conducted myself on set. She'd left the television network and launched her own production company, and didn't even think twice when it was time to hire a makeup artist.

It's been more than three years, and she has relocated out

of state, but I'm still her first call for makeup. We traveled and dined together, stayed in hotels where we had late-night girl talks and shared personal experiences, but when we hit the set, it was all business. Now, I didn't share this story to toot my own horn but to testify that someone's always watching.

Artist Tip

- **Do your job, remain professional and exercise discretion, regardless of what others in the industry do. Believe me, it will sustain you, because even when you think no one is paying attention - they are.**

Another artist tip comes to mind here: Don't become so cozy with your colleagues that it interferes with your job performance. Know your boundaries. Although we may hang out from time to time, she's still my superior, and I'm expected to deliver a professional service.

Being a freelance artist full-time is HARD. You have to hustle to get your name on the list of prospective clients, and even then, people forget about you. It's constantly reaching out to follow up with those you've worked with and amassed along the journey. There are a lot of gigs in the industry - we have to decide which ones to pursue, then put in the work to remain relevant.

During my early years, I applied for everything. Some gigs I loved, some I hated, but passion was always my driving force. You can tell the artists who are in it for the money, fame and opportunity to fellowship with famous people; they lack passion. During slow seasons, the ones without passion fall off, reverting back to their former careers, or embarking upon new ventures. Freelancing is either feast or famine; each season is unpredictable. Sometimes, I'm forced to decline offers because I'm already booked and sometimes, my phone doesn't ring.

Hello? Is anybody there? Is my phone working?

Once I got my foot in the door, I received calls for gigs around town, as well as some in Los Angeles. Most of the work I performed as a contractor at home was for BET Television. At BET, I met some incredible colleagues, as well as talent. Working as a contractor with the network was an amazing opportunity, which afforded me the opportunities of a lifetime. It was there I was able to hone my craft and learn about the entertainment industry. It was where I began to grow up and *glow up*.

My first big break came in January 2009. I was leaving my freelance shift at a department store cosmetics counter, when I noticed I had a message from a New York phone number. The caller wanted to know if I was available for an upcoming event in D.C. Although the caller didn't elaborate on the details, from the message I assumed this was a big deal. When I called her back to confirm my availability, I bubbled with excitement as the details unraveled. She didn't disclose the nature of the event, but I immediately discerned the job had something to do with the election of our first black president - Barack Obama!

Well, a week later, it was confirmed: I was hired as the makeup artist for the inaugural celebration concert. I was even asked to bring along an assistant. An assistant? I was ecstatic! All my hard work had paid off - now I was adding a substantial event to my résumé.

When I was advised of the celebrity lineup, I was in awe.

T.I., Tatiana Ali, Kerry Washington, Nick Cannon, and my boyfriend in my head - Common, amongst others.

When he arrived home that evening, I nearly tackled my husband to tell him the mind-blowing news that I would be grooming my boyfriend-in-my-head. (The side-eye he gave me is etched in my memory forever).

The concert was a tremendous success! Being the sole makeup artist came with perks. I groomed some of the industry's biggest stars, and was a part of history - President Obama's inauguration was all the rave! Afterwards, I was elated to book a gig for a group of pundits and reporters for BBC News. One of the most remarkable gigs was grooming those who would be covering the Inaugural Ball.

After being on set for ten hours, one of the reporters happened to drop in the bureau where I was stationed, requesting a makeup favor. She realized it was a last-minute request, but she wanted to be stunning for the ball. Of course, I obliged without giving it a second thought.

Now my hubby and I had already booked a trip to London for a course I was taking there. On the plane, he pointed to the television screen. My mouth fell to the floor when I saw the same reporter who'd asked a favor, covering the ball. She was gorgeous in her svelte gown, but I couldn't stop staring at her face. Knowing she'd been made up by me, I swelled with pride. I had no idea she'd be covering the festivities, I simply made sure she looked her best. Consider my day *made*.

Seeing my work on the big screen made me realize entertainment was the area I wanted to pursue. Film and television is a whole different ball game from retail beauty. This statement should be the artist's tip, because many makeup artists believe because they work in retail beauty, they can automatically transition to film and television. Slow your roll, and get proper training. All makeup applications are not created equal; I will be the first to attest that I thought the same. While in London, I was inspired and optimistic. I was excited by the course that I took. The artists abroad were so much more advanced, and more importantly - they were more forthcoming with information and advice.

The lessons I learned have shaped my career and the way I approach art. Namely, reaching the decision to create my own cosmetic line was a direct inspiration from my week abroad. Although I was taught about private labels in makeup school, it wasn't a desire of mine. However, being in a foreign place, surrounded by greatness, gave me a burst of creative drive I'd never experienced. I was reborn! After the rebirth, I committed to researching private label products, and how I could marry it with my freelance career.

Back home, a friend suggested I go for it. I wasn't sure if I wanted to at first, but being among the many different products, tools, books and incredible artistry made my spirit leap.

Game ON!

Although it took years to manifest my vision, that week was the jumpstart and the kick in the rear I needed to think beyond and ahead.

Blink

I left corporate America in 2005.
The following year, I was working with senators, actors, news anchors and television personalities. Whenever my schedule allowed, I freelanced in retail, because the gigs weren't steady. Remember: Working in this industry is feast or famine.

Sometimes my phone didn't ring; other times my hectic schedule forced me to decline bookings (I hate when that happens). All in all, I kept grinding. I was selected, rejected and neglected, but I kept going. Although being rejected did not feel good, it built my character for what was to come.

I will never forget the time I was being considered for a major ad with an agency.

I worked hard on developing my portfolio, and you should

have seen the leather attaché case I had purchased for the interview - it set me back a week's wages! My best work was displayed in the case, and I sashayed into the plush, upscale office both nervous and confident. I had no idea how this was going to turn out, but I was going to do my best.

When my appointment came up, I handed the owner of the agency my sleek portfolio. It was so awkward watching as she silently leafed through the pages with a stern face. She closed the book, bluntly dishing out her critique. Her assessment? My work was dated and restrictive. "No one does makeup like that anymore," she snapped.

I was devastated!

She went on to admonish me to study the makeup application in certain publications and magazines. I felt dismissed. With my throat filled with lumps and my heart in my lap, I mustered up the fortitude to thank her for the interview and advice. As I collected my bruised ego from the marble floor and prepared to make a quick exit with what was left of my dignity, she stopped me with a wave of the hand.

"That does not mean we can't use your talent."

Did I hear her correctly?

She extended her hand and welcomed me to the agency. I was placed on the new artist intake list, and my very first booking was a five-page spread for *Washington Life Magazine*! This was a huge deal - new artists were usually given menial tasks and assignments (perhaps with children or as an assistant), with seasoned artists. I was elevated before I got started!

The models were male, the venue elaborate and well beyond my pay grade. The director fell in love with me. From that day forward, she made sure I was booked for other gigs. I booked magazine shoots and television spots, as well as a few less prestigious assignments, but each one was worth it. On every single assignment, my nerves were off the charts, but I squared my shoulders and strolled on set with my game face. As far as they knew, I was a seasoned pro, and that's exactly how I behaved.

I didn't have much experience with male grooming, especially for print, so the initial shoot stressed me bad. Novice artists tend to believe applying men's makeup is easier, or should be approached the same as women's application. Sometimes, I think it's more difficult. The next few years found me in the throes of male grooming and doing makeup for print as well as film. I blinked, and three years had flown by! When you love what you do, it doesn't seem like work.

The year 2009 was remarkably busy for me and possibly the most pivotal one of my career. It was filled with many tremendous firsts: the first black president tops the list. I'll never forget being a part of such a monumental event. I arrived at the BBC to begin my day when the client informed me that the talent wouldn't arrive until several hours later. In a split second, I decided to leave my kit and walked the several blocks to the National Mall, to watch the swearing in of President Barack Obama. The energy was bananas! People walked the streets, cheering, greeting one another, high-fiving and simply relishing in the excitement. The camaraderie and unity was exhilarating and infectious. Blacks, whites and every other ethnicity was represented; in that moment of time, we were unified. Bring back those days; PLEASE!

As I stood freezing in record low temperatures taking in the incredible scene, a sense of pride and exhilaration that I could accomplish anything washed over me. That year was filled with major accomplishments. My schedule was booked, and my résumé was being stacked. I was on a roll!

I must've done something right when I worked the concert, because the next month I was booked for a hot gospel competition. Little did I know when I accepted the offer, that concert would be the first of many gospel shows I would have the privilege to work on. One gig led to another and so on. That summer, I was one of two makeup artists to work a coveted gospel show. Being a Christian, I was familiar with most artists that I made up, and it was a privilege to groom those whose music I'd grown up listening to.

The show filmed the entire season in six days, with only two artists. We worked our butts off! Some of my most memorable moments occurred during my tenure on that show. I was blessed to be an artist for five seasons. My work ethic and favor opened the door to other shows, and working one-on-one with some of the recording artists.

I'll never forget the time I was booked to make up a super-hot artist for her birthday party, or the time I worked with an artist for the Super Bowl. I booked gigs in D.C., Los Angeles, New York, Virginia and Pennsylvania, working with recording artists, athletes, actors, actresses, news anchors, politicians and reality stars. I've been both pleasantly surprised and sorely disappointed by some of my clients. There are some I've vowed to never work with again, likewise, there have been personalities who were extremely pleasant and warm.

There was one particular talent who invited me to her hotel room after working together. When my assistant and I came in, she had laid out this gorgeous jewelry on a long table. She invited us to take whatever we wanted; the tags were still attached. My assistant was bashful and hesitant, while I proceeded to select a few items I wanted. Hey - if she insisted, who was I to disappoint? Those were some nice pieces.

Four years later, she was planning a wedding in the Caribbean, and contacted me for makeup. She secured lodging and travel arrangements, a year in advance. I was stunned when she called to inform me the wedding was canceled. Before I could offer my condolences, she blew me away:

"I want you and your husband to go on vacation, and it's on me."

What?!?!

The more I protested the generous gift, the more insistent she became. "It's already been paid for," she said. "I've informed the hotel not to ask for your credit card at any time."

I couldn't believe what I heard. We accepted the vacation, and had an incredible time. I felt guilty she wasn't getting married and we were vacationing on her dime, but I enjoyed seven days of paradise. This is merely a sample of the blessings I've experienced over the years. It's been quite remarkable; the many successes as well as lessons which have come along the way. I don't count my shortcomings or disappointments as losses, only lessons.

One such lesson came when I was hired for a show by two different producers, each of whom had their own celebrity talent. I was to make up the first celebrity, then head over a few blocks away to make up the second one. A car was sent to transport me to the second location, relieving me of the stress of not having enough travel time.

I finished the first talent, who was a major B Lister. When

Mayvis Payne

I finished her makeup, she liked it, but called a relative (who was not a makeup artist), to get her approval. She facetimed the relative, who criticized my work as *too much,* adding that the color was off, as well. Now I knew the makeup was spot on, but that stung like a slap in the face.

With the adage, "the customer is always right" at the forefront of my mind, I asked what she would like to change. Keep in mind, I should've been packing my kit to relocate to the next destination, but customer service matters, not my feelings or expertise. I needed to ensure she was happy. Her relative recommended that I wipe most of the makeup off, which I happily obliged. Oh - did I mention this was a televised red-carpet event?

But, back to my story.

I wiped off the makeup per her request; however, I internally groaned. I knew it would look a hot, boiling mess on film and the red carpet, but that's what she wanted.

Traveling to the next client, I second-guessed my application and skills. She was a huge celebrity, yet one of the most pleasant talents I've ever worked with, even coming from a celebrity family, being constantly surrounded by staff and handlers. When I finished her face, she and her assistant marveled at my work, exclaiming it was the best she'd ever looked. I packed up my kit, took photos with her and some of the others and dashed to the venue for the taping.

Throughout the night, I was uneasy as I attended the show and after-show events. I even bumped into the first client at the after party, who spoke as though we were besties. I was cordial, but pretty much dismissed her and ventured to the other side of the room. Afterwards, I arrived at my hotel room, wondering how I could've been so far off with her makeup.

As I settled in for the night, I called my hubby. He knew the clients I was hired for, so he scoured social media for photos of the event. After making sure I was alright, he asked if I'd done Client A's makeup. He stumbled across photos of her, and noticed her makeup (or lack of) didn't look like my work. When I told him what happened, he assured me it was her call, and not to be bothered. That settled me down a little, although I was still rattled. This taught me an important lesson: I may have been the expert, but the client has the final say. It doesn't matter that I thought she needed more makeup; my goal is to satisfy the client - even if it's at my own demise.

When contracting for a network, artists truly have little control over what we can do or say. There have been times when clients have sat in my chair after having done their own makeup (which I had deemed to be horrendous), asking me to not remove it and just touch up their lips or eyes instead, and I've had to grin and bear it. I cringed when the show aired, seeing how horrible it looked on screen. This has caused me not to judge fellow artists' work harshly. Remember the next time you read a makeup artist's name in the credits, what you see may have been beyond their control.

Another lesson I've learned is to apply foundation first for live tapings - the direct opposite of what I was taught working retail. We were admonished to concentrate on the eyes first, so when the eye shadow falls onto the face, it won't be such a pain to clean. If foundation is already applied, it had to be wiped off and reapplied, which is an unnecessary, extra step. For years, this was my technique until....

During a live taping, a production assistant brought the client to makeup and said there was forty-five minutes until call time. This gave me the impression I could take my time - a rarity in live tapings. I began the application (eyes first), and had barely finished when the assistant burst in the room.

"She has to go," she said.

I was bewildered. At best, it had only been five minutes. "I thought I had more time; she's not finished."

"I'm sorry," she insisted, "but she has to be on stage, now!"

I was livid. The client only had eyeshadow - no foundation, lip products, blush, or false lashes. Who goes on television without lashes?

When the show aired, I was disappointed, but it wasn't as bad as I expected. Thankfully, she was young, and had fantastic skin. To this day, I apply at least a sheer layer of foundation first...just in case.

Artist Tip

- **Have a backup plan for the unexpected, especially for live tapings and performances. It will save a lot of stress.**

Blades, Shades & Charades

If there's one regret I have about my career, it's the backstabbing and dishonesty I've witnessed in this industry. I've always heard the term cutthroat, but I found out just what it meant firsthand.

Ironically, the greatest pain I've suffered came from those whom I introduced and helped get recognition and opportunities in the industry. Rule number one? Don't give your business card to people when you're working as an assistant or subbing for another artist. I've encountered this mess one too many times, each time blown away by the callous disrespect of other artists. Being unaware is one thing, but I've seen seasoned artists do it, too.

One summer, a colleague begged me to take her along as my assistant on a show I was booked for. She'd never worked outside of retail, and wanted a chance to work on a show. After some consideration, I decided to give her a shot. She was totally green, so I made sure to give her a rundown of the do's and don'ts on set, and industry conduct. On the first day, she failed the test miserably. As we neared the end of a long fourteen-hour day, one of the stagehands pulled me aside because the assistant distributed her business card to most of the staff and guests. I never saw her with cards, so it was clear she handed them out when I wasn't around or paying attention. As soon as we got in my car, I asked her about it. She confessed, but assured me she'd only given a card to a certain person. She claimed she didn't recall me mentioning it was wrong, so I questioned why she did it secretly if that were the case. She didn't have an answer. That's when I confronted her about asking the producer if she could work additional days. Thank God the producer instructed her to ask me, but she never got the chance; I fired her right on the spot.

That wasn't the last time I was stabbed in the back – there were more occasions. *Many* more, actually.

Shortly after the previous incident, I got a friend booked for a multi-day shoot. I found out exactly how much of a friend she really was. She resided out of state, so I opened our home to her to prevent her from spending money for a hotel. Not only did I get her booked and provide lodging, I cooked her breakfast every morning before we left for the show. A few months later, do you know how she repaid me?

She called the producer (whom I introduced her to), saying she had makeup artist friends who'd like to work on her shows, so they didn't have to book *me* all the time. Yep, you read that right! Now, remember she lived out of state and so did the other artists. She wanted the producer in my state to decline my services and hire her friends in another state.

Delete. Unfriend. CANCEL.

The producer never hired her again. And might I add, her first high-profile job was booked off a referral from ME, followed by multiple bookings on another show, again - based on my referral. We're talking tens of thousands of dollars, the opportunity to make a name for herself and many more chances to build her résumé with celebrity clientele and projects. And that's how she thanked me. To date, she no longer gets booked for high-profile gigs. I hope it was well worth it. Sayonara!

Another example comes to mind.

Once while in retail, I assisted a young lady and her mother with their makeup application. As I did their makeovers, we chatted a bit about my life as a makeup artist. The daughter aspired to be an industry artist herself, noting that her mother worked for a major television network. We exchanged information and they left after purchasing their products. Months later, I received a text from the daughter asking if I was available to work two days on a temporary project. She said she'd previously worked with the production coordinator, but couldn't work on this project because she worked full-time in another profession. I accepted the invitation, and she passed my contact information onto the production coordinator. I ended up getting booked beyond the two days I was contracted for. The crew loved working with me and I was invited to work an extended period.

Because I knew this referral was connected to the young lady, I reached out to her to inquire whether she'd like the opportunity instead. She assured me work obligations kept her from accepting the gig, and encouraged me to continue. She also admitted she didn't have much experience, and if the opportunity arose, she'd love to shadow me on future projects. I told her I'd keep her in mind when the opportunity to bring an assistant along became available.

We remained in contact, and I discovered she had minimal experience, therefore I was eager to help. A few months later, I was hired for a show and was asked to bring an assistant. I immediately thought of her, and invited her to come along. I explained the terms along with the pay rate, to which she agreed. Over the next couple of weeks, I expressed my expectations to her, including conduct, rules of the trade, and asked about her kit. She assured me that her kit was film-friendly and I felt confident to have her assist me.

On filming day, we agreed to commute together on the train. I was taken aback when I laid eyes on her unprofessional attire. With her mother working for a major network, I expected her to be abreast of television culture, including wardrobe. I shrugged it off, though it made me uneasy.

The show was a talent competition, and the guests were a mixture of contestants and celebrity judges. As the contestants arrived, I noticed her bubbly disposition fading. There were only the two of us, so I split the talent evenly. As I worked on my first female client, I glanced at the one in her chair, and stopped dead in my tracks. Her application was so horrendous, in order to fix it, the client's face needed to be cleaned and started from scratch. We were on a strict timetable, so I completed my person and made up an excuse to have her talent sit in my chair. I decided to have her make up the male contestants instead, and she said she was comfortable with it.

But when I asked to see her products, that's when I *knew*.

She was way out of her league. Every single item in her kit was all wrong for television or film. What was I going to do? Not only had I taken on the bulk of the talent, but now I had to provide her with the proper products and guide her through each application on top of that. All of this without letting anyone know what was happening. Thankfully, the show was running hours behind schedule.

When the celebrity judge arrived, I went to his suite and groomed him. After I was done, I told him I would introduce him to my assistant, and she'd be the one to pat him down if he perspired. Nothing else needed to be done; he was good for the entire taping. He was fine with that, so I went to get her. I gave her the necessary products for touch-ups, and introduced them so I could return to the makeup room to finish up the remaining contestants. When I checked in on her, I noticed she seemed awfully giddy and doe-eyed. I walked her outside, where she expressed how cute she thought the talent was. I reminded her about onset conduct, and instructed her to return to the makeup room until he called.

As the day went on, I noticed she went missing. When I checked in on the celebrity guest, I found her in his suite. Earlier when I introduced them, I whispered to her to be sure to get a photo with him for her portfolio. She'd never heard of him and had no clue how famous he was, but I understood the importance of building a strong résumé and portfolio. Besides, I remembered the feeling when I worked with my first celebrity; I wanted that memory for her.

When I popped in, she was giggling, cozying up to him and snapping multiple selfies. I didn't know if he was offended or flattered, but he informed us he was planning to close the door and chill until taping began, so we left him alone. She and I got through the day and went our separate ways. A couple of weeks later, I saw her tagging him on her social media page, commenting that if he ever needed a makeup artist to reach out to her. I mean she inserted ALL her contact information.

That did it.

I reached out asking to have a conversation, but she claimed she wasn't available to chat. Since she was dodging me, I sent a flurry of text messages. First, I sent an event recap, offering suggestions on what could've been done differently. Next, I expressed my thoughts regarding her on-set conduct, lack of preparation, as well as the comments on the client's social media page. I was already a follower of his because I'd worked with him on a couple of other occasions; however, I never commented, messaged or even asked to work with him again. He remembered me, said it was great to see and work with me again, and I left it at that. I have discovered, if an artist or talent wants to work with you again, they'll ask for your information and contact you - which has happened to me on several occasions. Most of the time the network hires the crew anyway, and the talent has little input on who's hired.

She was HOT. She said she didn't appreciate me telling her how to conduct herself, and that she should've gotten paid more, even though I paid her far beyond what I was ever paid as an assistant. Eventually, she blocked me on social media and I never heard from her again.

Because of this and various other instances, my vetting process has improved drastically over the years; however, I'm still somewhat leery of hiring assistants. Now if she were asked, she might say I was jealous, insecure etc., but none of that applies to me. We should always remain professional with talent and never get too comfortable. Period. They're not friends, colleagues or associates – they are clients. This is how I conduct myself on set, and I make sure my assistants follow suit. I was taught to follow the leader; if they don't do it, neither should you. Besides, we discussed conduct prior to the event, so there was no excuse.

...which reminds me of another occurrence. Sheesh, I might need a Volume 2!

Early in my career, I was booked for one gig, and requested for another the same day. The second gig was simple enough, so I asked if I could send my assistant. The production company agreed, and booked her. Weeks later, I met with the hairstylist who worked the gig where my assistant attended. During our conversation, she mentioned having never seen a makeup artist arrive on set with a bare face.

I was livid!

"Do you mean to tell me she arrived without wearing makeup?" I asked.

"Yes," she replied casually, "and everyone noticed it."

I couldn't wait to get to my phone. I called the assistant, confronting her about what I'd been told. She shrugged it off, saying she didn't like wearing makeup.

"You're representing me," I fussed. "How many times have you seen me arrive on set without makeup?"

"None," she quipped (displaying a major attitude).

And NONE is the exact number of times she ever substituted for me again.

A couple of years ago, I was working on a week-long shoot

from hell, and the stylist was accompanied by two assistants. One of them arrived late on the very first day, which resulted in a mad dash to get all of the talent suited and transported to the off-site set.

Did I mention it was a shoot from hell?

Throughout the week, the lead kept pulling one of the assistants to the side, and the look on her face said she was unhappy with his direction. Every day, she was either tardy, ignoring his instructions, or goofing up the wardrobe. On the last day of the shoot, I walked to get a cup of coffee and when I got back, I was startled to see her leaving the building. She hadn't arrived when we checked in, so I cheerfully greeted her at the door. When she didn't respond, I chalked it up to her not hearing me.

On the set, I discovered she'd been fired. Too many missed opportunities to learn, glean and grow - it didn't have to be that way.

Artist Tip

- **Always remember that you are your brand (or a representative of someone else's). Everything you do and say represents you or them, therefore present yourself well. And, if you are subbing for or assisting another artist, take their cue and follow their lead. A huge part of being a great assistant is researching the lead artists' conduct, personality and demeanor, not solely their skill.**

- **As a newbie, don't be so stubborn to do things your own way. Learn from those who've come before you. Seasoned artists may not have all of the answers, but our clients trust that we know what we're doing.**

Looking Glass

I was once asked why I continue working with brides, prom girls, etc., while being a makeup artist to the stars. The answer is simple - everyone is a star in my chair! Why should it matter who the client is? Every face deserves your best brush forward.

For one thing, most celebrities change makeup artists frequently; it's easier to find a stylist in the city where they'll be performing, and most of us don't have the luxury of traveling with the rich and famous. Even if I did travel with my clients full-time, when my schedule permits, I'd still offer my services to those who aren't famous. Why? Because I love what I do, and I love seeing faces enhanced. I love the look on a client's face after they receive my special treatment. More importantly, I never want to forget my humble beginnings.

Mayvis Payne

Although I don't believe I have "arrived," I'm in awe and eternally grateful to God for affording me the opportunity to live out my wildest dreams. I've worked with some of the industry's biggest names, traveled to places I never thought I would visit, worked and played in some of the most beautiful arenas and homes I've ever seen.

I've been told my résumé is impressive. Sometimes, my accomplishments surprise me, just as much as others. I've come a long way, and have often forgotten some of the projects that I've worked on. Once, I heard a familiar voice on television. When I looked up, I was surprised to see a commercial that I had worked on. The rush I felt was more than exhilarating! Moments like these are priceless.

Although our vocation looks easy, it is far from it; that is the backstory that is often overlooked. I've had to put in some hard work. I've been rejected, sneered at and I have had friends and colleagues stab me in the back. My calls have sometimes been ignored and dismissed, but I have persevered and ultimately succeeded.

There are countless stories that can't be revealed in this book, but I hope to always remain humble and never think of myself more highly than I am. Everyone deserves beauty. It shouldn't matter how rich or how famous you are or are not.

Shame on me if I snub someone for not being famous or wealthy. Furthermore, I didn't get to where I am on my own - there were many people who supported me in some shape or form. There were those who encouraged me, referred me, gave me a chance or recognized my potential. Even with the odds stacked against me, God always granted me favor, and a door eventually swung open. I can't help but reflect on how this little chick from Mississippi made her way to the Big Apple. Who would've thought it? I wonder if my grandmother saw it in me as she was teaching me life lessons without even knowing.

When I was young, I watched as my aunts and uncles went off to pick cotton, which was a high paying job back then. I begged my grandmother to allow me to go and become the "water girl", but she always said no. That alone was traumatizing, because my grandparents pretty much let me have my way...but I'm off topic.

Each time they prepared to leave, I asked her again, hoping to change her mind. I'd already calculated the money I'd make if she'd just say yes, that's why I kept right on asking. And she kept right on saying No; shooting me down every time.

I never understood why, because as far back as I can recall, Grams gave me carte blanche. Being the firstborn grandchild had its perks! But, not in those moments.

One day, she asked if I'd like to accompany her to her job as a domestic worker, cleaning homes and apartments for well-to-do white women. I cheerfully replied, "Yes!"

I absolutely loved spending time with my grandmother, a quiet storm. She didn't talk much, and rarely raised her voice (total opposite of me); however, she had a quiet resolve and exuded the kind of peace that made anyone comfortable.

Due to emotional trauma (another book for another time), I don't remember much about my childhood, but I vividly recall conversations with my grandmother as I helped her make beds or relaxing as she hot-combed my long, thick hair, or while helping her hang laundry on the clothesline in the backyard. She never judged me, at least not out loud. She listened intently to my heart, and responded in love; sometimes scolding me, but ever so gently. My Grams took me to church, taught me how to cook (I can throw down in the kitchen), instructed me in Scripture and taught me how to work hard with integrity.

Now that I think about it, it was no ordinary feat that she gained the trust of the women she worked for. Other than pictures in their homes, I never saw the ladies, because they trusted her with a key to come and go while they were away at work. I would watch as she traveled from room to room, meticulously cleaning each one to pristine perfection. She scrubbed toilets, mopped floors, cleaned ovens, changed linens, did the laundry, vacuumed and dusted. She would take a break midday and prepare lunch for her and me, making sure to wash the dishes and leave the kitchen spotless.

Sometimes, I would help with her tasks, and sometimes she worked alone, most likely to protect the boss's privacy. She even paid me sometimes, though I wasn't expecting it. I gleaned so much simply by observing her, and respected how she worked. Just being able to spend quality time with her was all the compensation I needed.

My grandparents married when they were incredibly young, and stayed together more than seventy years until my grandfather passed away from cancer. In addition to birthing and rearing fifteen biological children, they raised me for several years. I am the first-born grandchild, out of sixty-six grandchildren and to say that they spoiled me is an understatement.

Yep, you read that correctly: sixty-six! Shout-out to all of my cousins; hey y'all! See? Southern girl all the way.

Even when I lived with my mother, I spent most of my time at my grandparents' home. Not only did my grandmother clean other people's houses, her home remained spotless. She cooked everything from scratch, and we all ate dinner together at the dining table at five o'clock, when PawPaw came home from work. My grandmother always had a hot meal prepared, and we thoroughly enjoyed her delicious home-cooking. I can still taste those hot butter rolls, biscuits, upside-down pound cake, pot roast and many more dishes. She knew how to take very few items and make an enormous spread, with enough for second helpings. Additionally, there was always something sweet to top off dinner. She was a magician, I tell you - effortlessly making something out of nothing.

Occasionally, my grandparents loaded us into PawPaw's station wagon and took us to visit his relatives in the country. His relatives were so deep in the hills, they had out-houses instead of indoor bathrooms. (I still shudder thinking what could've been lurking around it). Once while visiting, my aunt went to the yard, selected a chicken, slaughtered it and fried it up. That was by far the best chicken and dressing I had ever tasted, but right out of the yard? Ewwwww!

So why am I mentioning all of this? Because it's important to my story. Sometimes our perceived success hinders us from failing to acknowledge the back story; the parts we wish to forget.

Those experiences have helped mold me into the person I am today. Peering into the looking glass every now and then keeps you grounded and helps put things into proper perspective – if you allow it. I've encountered and worked with famous people who have come from humble beginnings;

however, they treat the hired help like crap. Or they act high and mighty, as if they were reared with a silver spoon in their mouths. Even if that were the case, it's no reason to snub or look down your nose at anyone.

I recall once I groomed a former child star. As an adult, she wasn't as famous, but I was excited to work with her. She loved her makeup and wrote down the products that I used and asked for my social media accounts. Although she was no longer a huge star, she refused to follow me on IG, because she said I didn't have enough followers. Ma'am; have several seats!

Then, there was the time when a R&B star refused to ride the elevator with us, because we were too common. I know her story, she grew up in one of the roughest places in the world, came from a broken home and rose to stardom. Clearly, she had forgotten where she's come from. She is wonderfully talented, however that attitude has limited her success.

Once, I was summoned to work on a show in the Deep South. It had been several years since I'd been back, so I was excited to go, especially to discover how much the south had evolved. Who am I kidding? I was excited about the down-home cooking I planned to enjoy…and enjoy, I did!

I arrived at my hotel, settled in and enjoyed a few hours until the meet-and-greet with the celebrity talent, who was expected later that evening. As soon as I laid eyes on her, I knew she was going to be a handful. Unfortunately, I was right. Over the next few days, she managed to ruffle more than a few feathers. She wasn't a nice person at all! She'd recently undergone a major transformation, and she was doing the most. The funny thing is, no one really recognized *her*; they kept asking me and the other glam squad if we were famous. She wouldn't allow the limo driver to leave his post - he was instructed to sit in front of the hotel, so people would know someone important was there. I felt so bad for him. He and I hit it off, and I kept him company for a bit, passing time until we had to leave again. *By now you know I'm not shy...*

At breakfast one morning, I noticed one of the young ladies who worked at the hotel recognized *Miss Thang,* and made her way to the table with a pen and pad. Our eyes met, and I discreetly motioned *not now*, and she obliged. An hour later as we were preparing to walk out the door, the young lady came over to shoot her shot.

"Hello Miss - I'm a huge fan," she meekly said. "May I have your autograph please?" *Miss Thang* looked the sweet girl up and down, looked her in the eyes and spat, **"No!"**

I was flabbergasted; the young lady was visibly crushed.

She glared at me, clearly embarrassed, and all I could do was offer an apology with sympathetic eyes, because I was just as shell-shocked as she was. I'm sure the young lady will remember that humiliating incident for the rest of her life. Disgusting! I mean, we were exiting the building and we had plenty of time, so why not indulge a fan? But, as I discovered over the next few days, she was not partial. She was just as rude and unkind to the crew and set staff. Oh, the names she was secretly being called!

Another time, I was walking with friends to the elevator when we passed by a huge A-lister. Being fans of hers, my friends fell over themselves. Once they got brave enough to request a photo, she was incredibly rude.

"Here we go again," she huffed. "I'm only taking one picture - that's it. Good-bye!"

Mayvis Payne

My friends were so disgusted by her attitude, they vowed never to support her again.

That was almost ten years ago. One of my friends shared that she still can't bear to watch her on television, because of that one incident. It's true what they say: First impressions are important. How I wish all celebrities would remember that. Fans are responsible for creating a star; were it not for the fans, would you even become famous? I understand there are times they want to be left alone, but in this instance, she wasn't having dinner, out with her family, or in the middle of an interview. She was on her way out the door, so why not indulge her admirers with a quick photo or autograph - with a smile? It would have made someone's day.

Instances like these help me appreciate the kind, gentle, humble and genuine talents I've worked with. One celebrity who immediately comes to my mind is Mo Rocca. Mo is one of the most down-to-earth talents I've ever had the pleasure of working with.

I was referred to work on a show for the Cooking Channel, where Mo was the host. I'd heard of him, and because he's such a big star, I wasn't expecting what I encountered. Filming days were long, but he and the crew made it so easy, it didn't seem like work. Sometimes, we'd be on location, and passers-by recognized him, and called out, "Hey - that's Mo Rocca!" Mo stopped and engaged with them, complete with giggles, jokes and selfies.

In addition to his talent and humility, Mo is one of the funniest people I've ever met. He laughed with bystanders as if they were long lost friends; I've witnessed it on several occasions. He may have been exhausted, and some days I'm sure he wanted to just retreat to his hotel room, but you'd never know it by observing him. I was pleasantly surprised to discover just how easy it was to be around him because he's genuinely a nice guy. The first time I went to his home, Mo welcomed me as if I were a childhood pal. Years later, I still receive the same reception. Annually, the crew gathers for dinner to keep in touch, and it's magical. Not only do we get together to catch up, but we have inducted our spouses and family members. A huge shout-out to my fellow Raviolians…the best crew ever!

Piers Morgan was another celebrity who pleasantly surprised me. From his television persona, I was terrified as we were being introduced. He was the complete opposite of what I expected - he was warm and chatty, cracked jokes, asked about my stance on political agendas, and even invited me to dinner with the team. I declined; however, I was instantly enamored and garnered so much respect for him.

It's people like these and many others, who really raise the bar and make an artist's job so much more special. Whenever I encounter a difficult client, I try not to let it dampen my spirit. Instead, I remember one bad apple doesn't spoil the whole bunch.

My Grams taught me that. *Rest in peace Grams.*

I've also witnessed makeup artists, hairstylists and other glam professionals act haughty, simply because they're working with a celebrity. I've been shunned by some of those artists who thought they were better, more important or more famous.

Once while working on a show, the head of the makeup department wouldn't send any celebrity clients to my chair. I was hired directly by the network executives, which put her in her feelings. She didn't think I was skilled enough to work on the show, with the celebrity glam squad. To add insult to injury, I was getting paid twice as much as her team. How do I know? Because she asked if I would reduce my rate. A few years later, I was referring clients to her, because I was completely booked. This is a great time to mention that this is the same artist who had shunned me many years earlier, when I was trying to break into the business. But, even after all of that, I was not bitter; I still referred clients to her whenever possible...Because I know who I am.

There's a saying in the industry: You're only as good as your last assignment.

Just because you're working with a star today, doesn't guarantee you'll be with them for the long haul. You're no better than aspiring artists or new kids on the block. I've witnessed glam squads behave as if they're the talent, arriving late to set, and entering the room like *All hail the Queen (or King)*.

Puh-leez!

Don't be grand. We're employees, hired to provide a service, then step out of the way so the talent can shine.

Artist Tip

- **Don't ever forget: We are hired to provide a behind-the-scenes service, not to be in the spotlight.**
- **Remain humble and don't compare yourself to others. Just do you. If more artists understood this, backstabbing wouldn't be so prevalent in this industry.**

Exiting my soapbox...for now.

I've always shied away from the spotlight. The Bible says your gift will make room for you. We are to operate in the vocation for which we have a purpose, and if anything more comes of it, chalk it up to divine favor.

No need to exhaust yourself, trying to get to the top...what's meant for you is for YOU.

I'm reminded of working with a personality for an annual televised event. I had to remain with her on the red carpet, and green-room backstage. The room was filled with celebrities, handlers, assistants and network staff. I was the only glam artist present, because I was asked to accompany the talent. Most of the staff fell all over themselves trying to cozy up to a particular celebrity, who was loud, flirty and boisterous. A crowd gathered around him; however, I was completely turned off by his obnoxious behavior. Every other word was laced with profanity and nasty complaints about the quality of the food being served to us. I'm no prude, but I felt all the extra wasn't necessary. There was another young lady standing nearby, who seemed to be as unfathomed as me. We bumped into each other a couple of times, and exchanged pleasantries.

After a few minutes, we asked each other about our roles. It turned out she was the assistant to one of the biggest names on the show. We exchanged cards, and she bid me goodbye before turning to go out on the floor to her seat. When I told her I'd be watching the monitors from the back, she spun on her heels and asked if I needed a ticket.

Sidebar: The network was notorious for not providing tickets to the glam squad for the show, unless you were a part of the clique (which clearly, I was not). I've never been fond

Mayvis Payne

of cliques, but I should remain focused on the storyline...

Before I could answer, she pulled out an envelope filled with tickets. As she flipped through them, she said she couldn't give me one of the floor seats, but I was welcome to a seat in the back. I told her I didn't care where I sat- I was just grateful she offered.

We'd been backstage for an hour, and since my talent had already performed, there was no reason for me to stay backstage. No one paid us any attention, but as soon as she gave me that ticket and walked away, a couple of people ran over, asking me if she'd given me a ticket. "Yes," I cheerfully sang, "and it grants me access to the after party."

As I walked to the stage door, I was greeted by about four or five other celebrity glam artists. I wish you could've seen their faces when they saw me. They were sitting outside the stage door, trying to peek in to see the celebrity-packed show. One man's mouth hit the floor when he saw me. I felt the stares as I waltzed past them, said hello and handed the usher my ticket. She escorted me across the first row of seating, directly past celebrities who always get the best seats in the house, and rightfully so. I couldn't understand why she was taking me the long way around until she motioned to my seat.... in the third row! From the stage!

What?!?!

I couldn't believe it!

Karen - the assistant, had secretly given me a ticket to one of the best seats on the floor. I was surrounded by celebrities; heck, some of them were behind me. My seat was better than most of theirs! I will never forget the way one lady looked at me like, *Who is she*? I played it cool; however, I was shaking inside. I'm talking about shook!

Before I could wrap my mind around what had just transpired, my cell phone vibrated. *Thank God I keep my phone on silent when I'm at work.* I let it go to voicemail, then noticed a text message pop up on my screen. It was from a fellow celebrity makeup artist; one of those I'd passed backstage.

OMG! Are you on the floor? I see you on the screen!

YES, I discreetly responded to the text as I put my phone away and enjoyed the rest of the show. Once I regained my composure, I glanced down the row and caught the eye of my celebrity client, who gave me a thumbs-up.

I silently thanked God a million times. I'll never forget that moment and the kindness Karen showed me. I was mindful to send her a thank-you email, and I'm forever grateful for that opportunity.

Seven years earlier, I was starting off as an artist, and one of my friends gave me a ticket to attend a show as her guest. No one knew me and I didn't have celebrity clients. To top it off, my seat was on the very last row...of that very same theater...for the same show. Talk about coming full circle!

Stay in your lane and keep doing your best. Your gift will make room for you.

By far my most memorable client was the late Dr. Maya Angelou. She was so regal, her presence alone made me shiver. Royalty oozed from her very being. Talking with her was as if I were having a conversation with one of my aunts - so easy and familiar. When I entered her suite, I was extremely nervous; however, a single sentence from her calmed my nerves. *"Hello beautiful; and what is your name?"*

By far, Dr. Angelou was the largest presence on the roster,

Mayvis Payne

yet she took the time and asked questions about me. She was generally interested in knowing who I was; little ole me. Time stood still, especially as she poured out her wisdom into us while we waited backstage. There wasn't a dry eye to be found; everyone was crying. She was that elegant, wise and regal. I can't even read the term regal now, without thinking of her. Regal is who she was and yet is, even in death.

And to think I was the newest makeup artist on the show. The others had tenure and probably should've been selected over me; however, once again FAVOR prevailed. I'll never forget the PC whispering to me, "Get a kit together. I want you to go and groom Dr. Maya Angelou." My eyes bulged and my heart beat so fast, I thought it would jump right out of my chest. I had to use my hands to close my mouth, because it was frozen wide open. I'm grateful to that particular PC, for helping to orchestrate some of the most pivotal moments of my career. She always made sure I got the top names in my chair.

These experiences were many moons ago, but it's always good to look back, to gage how far you've come. I hope to always occasionally gaze in the mirror of life, so that I don't become too big for my britches (as Grams used to say).

Glitter and Grime

"*It must be so cool being a celebrity makeup artist.*" I've been told this more times than I can count.

The fact of the matter is, it's really cool being a makeup artist, PERIOD. No celebrity status required. Don't get me wrong, I've certainly had some amazing opportunities and met some of the most incredible people, but simply being able to earn a living doing what you love? That's what I call *glitter*.

We've all heard the mantra: People see your glory, but they don't know your story. Truer words have never been spoken. Most people don't consider the gutter experiences - those things which have marred the journey along the way. These are often the norm, not the exception. It's funny thinking how no one really approached me about being my assistant until my name was on the screen or attached to a particular project. I received no requests when I was navigating through the blood, sweat and tears. No one wanted any parts of that!

Was I a good makeup artist prior to my name being seen?

I suppose that's why people are always so shocked to learn of the failures that are a prelude to successes. Society has conditioned us to focus on the glitter. The truth is, the door has been slammed in my face one too many times, and my high hopes crushed on several occasions. But do you know what I did each time? Wallow, suck it up, then try again.

Let's talk about wallowing for a moment. We rarely want to discuss that part as we struggle to maintain contrived smiles, feigning joy along the journey; however, that's not my testimony. I've struggled and waded through difficult days. I cried, second-guessed myself, wondered whether I should return to corporate, asked God why (and why not), and even doubted whether becoming a makeup artist was the right decision. The one thing I haven't done? BEG. Nope, not gonna do it!

I still recall one of my most poignant heartbreaks. It cut me so deep, the pain is still fresh. It doesn't hurt anymore, but I still recall how it made me feel. I worked with the producer of a major production for several years. I thought we had a rather good rapport, but now I realize it was all business…shady business.

When we first met, I was new to the business, which she used to her advantage. As time went on and I began learning more, I noticed a change in her interactions with me. I became cognizant regarding my role and started requesting certain amenities and allowances.

In the beginning, she seemed to trust me so much, and even booked me for her own company, in addition to hiring me for the major production. Eventually, she grew less cordial towards me, especially when we were on set, even though I'd done makeovers for her, her family, friends, colleagues, etc. Once, she even asked me to lie to her boss if he approached me about something she'd done! (She should be thankful he never asked). Anyway, there were tons of times when she quoted a lower than standard rate. Of course, I knew, but I was building my résumé and getting loads of experience, so I didn't mind – I thought we had each other's back.

I worked several annual shows, so I never thought twice when one of them was scheduled to begin filming, expecting her to call me with the schedule. One of the crew members I referred called when he noticed my name wasn't listed on the crew roster. You read correctly: my recommendation was booked, I was not. There had to be some type of mistake.

I reached out to the producer, who initially ignored my call. She finally responded that she was no longer booking crew, and that I needed to contact her subordinate. I did as instructed, and he responded, "We already have our crew." No explanation, no formal complaints, no consideration, nothing. Now this may seem trivial, but I was crushed. Not only had I bent over backwards for her, but I referred a lot of people who were eventually hired for her shows.

I'd attended parties at her home, we traveled together, dined together, and I always worked within the confines of her budget, with the presumption that we were mutually connected, so crushed is an understatement.

Several people contacted me, inquiring why I wasn't on the

roster, and a couple of celebrity guests called complaining about their makeup application and why wasn't I there? I didn't have a good answer, because I was clueless about what happened myself. I wallowed in self-pity, wondering what I'd done wrong. I'll never forget standing at my bathroom sink with tears in my eyes when I heard the Holy Spirit's voice:

"Why are you concerned about the fish in the pond, when I've given you the ocean?"

I wish I could tell you I immediately knew what those words meant or that I was instantly encouraged, but it didn't happen that way. All I can say is I continued pursuing other leads, cold-calling, sharing my résumé, and networking...I kept going. Wounded, but mobile. *Ooooo, that could be another book title! An author is being birthed....*

Eventually, I began to snag more mainstream opportunities with bigger budgets, which led to more substantial projects. I didn't even apply for these gigs; people were requesting me left and right. I went from being told what the project's budget was to being asked what was my rate. The stars were bigger than I'd ever worked with before, and I started traveling with the cast and crew. Before I knew it, my résumé swelled so much, I had to hire a résumé-writer, booking agent and marketing professional.

Succinctly, I was swimming in the ocean.

While I was healing from the previous incident, I encountered another memorable celebrity interaction, and not in a good way.

I was booked for a series, and when I researched the talent, something about her profile told me she is going to be difficult to work with.

Sidebar: I intensely research the talent prior to working with them.

Artist Tip

- **Be sure to do your due diligence - it helps tremendously.**

I had heard this celebrity's name before, but had never worked with her or knew anyone who had. Once again, my discernment was spot on. Henceforth, we will refer to her as DT – or, *Difficult Talent*.

DT strolled into the green room, cold and standoffish, at least towards me. She was buddies with the rest of the crew, and she made sure I was aware that I was only hired because her personal makeup artist was unavailable for the day. Eventually, her makeup artist was only available once or twice during the series, therefore I ended up being the regular artist for several months (yay me!). Each session, DT directed me how to apply her makeup. If I did anything to her liking, she wouldn't say a word, but was extremely vocal when she didn't like it. The makeup she preferred was not flattering or appropriate for television, so I was caught in a really tough conundrum.

One morning, she was to interview another celebrity guest, and I was assigned to groom them both. When I tell you she performed, please believe it!

She belittled my application, loud enough for the entire room to hear. According to her, the foundation color was off, she hated the lipstick, the lashes weren't dramatic enough, and she needed more blush. Basically, nothing I did was good enough for her. Never mind the fact this was probably my 20th time doing her makeup, and the foundation had never changed. That being said, the customer is always right, correct?

Mayvis Payne

Prior to her arrival, I had completed the celebrity guest's makeup and she loved it so much, she asked if she could write down everything I used on her. But after the homegirl's tirade, the guest's body language changed; she wasn't as friendly as she was earlier. The air in the green room was extremely tense and the guest and her assistant cowered in the corner to themselves.

Once we got on set, DT turned it up a few notches. Every few minutes, she called for me to touch her up. The hairstylist was nowhere in sight, so that left me with double duty. I glanced at the guest a few times and her eyes told me all I needed to know. Her responses were short, she was grimacing and arms were folded, as if she wanted to be anywhere but there.

Between the touch up marathon, the snarky remarks and verbal abuse directed towards me, I was totally drained by the time we wrapped. I don't think I even said goodbye, I just packed up my kit, grabbed my coat and left.

I ran into one of DT's friends on my way out. Apparently, my face said it all. She tried to assure me DT treated everyone she likes in that manner, and if she didn't like me, I wouldn't be there. She tried to justify the bad behavior by informing me that DT had major connections and many pending opportunities I could benefit from, by being on her team.

Whew, chile - I wasn't having it! I told her I don't tolerate abuse from anyone, no matter who they are. We said our goodbyes and I made my way to the train station, fuming all the way home.

I didn't know how, but the situation had to be handled.

The next day, I was booked for another show. On my break,

I called the producer from the series, venting about the mess from the day before. I told her that I wouldn't tolerate that type of behavior from the DT anymore, and was assured that the producer would handle it. By the way, I absolutely adored this producer. Years earlier, she observed me working on another show, and when she got the opportunity to have her own, she hired me. I really miss her.

Anyway, a couple of hours later, I received a call from one of the producers of the series. Due to me being booked that day on another gig, they hired another makeup artist because again, DT's personal makeup artist wasn't available. Well, DT was throwing a tantrum, because according to her, this makeup artist didn't know how to apply makeup and her kit was amateur. She was screaming in the background as the producer spoke to me. Guess what I heard her say?

"Where is Mayvis? If Mayvis can't be here tomorrow, I'm not coming!"

I mean, she yelled to the top of her lungs, hurling words I can't write here, but I'm sure you can use your imagination. When I returned the next day, she had nothing but good things to say about my ability to do beautiful makeup (her words; not mine). Suddenly, my approach to color mixing was superb, her eyeshadow was stunning, and I was the consummate professional. She even pulled out her phone and introduced me to her Periscope followers. She never gave me any more problems, although for whatever reason, the series ended up getting canceled. A couple of months later, the producer called me, reporting that DT requested my number.

"Should I give it to her?" She asked.

"Nah, I'll pass," I replied.

Mayvis Payne

Dang! It seems DT's personal makeup artist was never available.

Knowing my personality, the situation could've played out differently. I assure you I wanted so badly to give her a piece of my mind; however, I understood my assignment and felt it best to let the executives handle it. Besides, someone passing by or unaware of the circumstances would've thought I was the instigator. I could have been labeled unprofessional, difficult or rude. I never want to cause an environment to be hostile or tense, even when I'm fuming inside.

In the end, I won.

Artist Tip

- **Always maintain your composure and conduct yourself in a professional manner. Don't allow anyone to pull you into their negative energy. Take a step back and wait it out. Remember celebrities are people, just like you and me. They experience trauma, have bad days, get cranky, tired or are just plain rude. Whatever the case, don't lose your career over it.**

Speaking of uncomfortable environments…

I was hired to do makeup for a rap video. Six males were in the group; the lead artist had seen my work while in the studio with a photographer. I arrived on set, only to discover they were very much behind schedule. The lead artist assured me I'd be compensated for their tardiness, so I settled in and set up my station. When the band members started arriving, they reeked of marijuana and alcohol.

94

In a separate room, a table with every type of alcohol you can name was set up. As I began rotating the guys in for their grooming, I noticed the studio getting overcrowded. There were six ladies in the room and twenty men, excluding group members. The lead artist was last to be groomed; he came into my suite and paid me handsomely for my work, generous tip included. He told me I was finished for the day, but could stick around for the recording.

The music was blasting and party jumping, but I thanked him and headed home. I never leave before the production ends in case retouches are needed, but this time, I didn't think twice. Something felt off to me. It was getting late and I lived hours away, so I packed my things, said my goodbyes and rolled out.

A few days later, I reached out and thanked him for retaining my services. When I asked how the shoot went, he confessed it went horribly wrong. A fight broke out before filming was complete, and someone was shot!

He said he was glad I left when I did – the incident happened immediately after I left. Heck, I probably hadn't even made it to the expressway. That was my warning: never be so star-struck that you jump at any opportunity to mingle or rub elbows. Situations like these dissuade me from becoming too chummy with every celebrity client I meet.

Once after a long day on set, I retreated to the restaurant next door. I sat at the bar and ordered my food, while enjoying the solitude of the empty restaurant. The owner recognized me from filming on the street with the celebrity talent. Since he was a fan, he comped my tab and introduced me to the staff. As I ate, the celebrity I was working with came in with his team and the rest of the production crew. They all sat together and motioned for me to join them, but I responded I was finishing my dinner and heading home. The next day's call time was super early, so I had good reason to leave. When I arrived home and shared the story with my husband, he wondered whether it would be considered rude that I didn't join them.

I'd been hired for one day, but ended up working with them for the next two and a half weeks. I don't know how they felt about me declining the dinner invitation, but I choose to believe my professionalism played a major part in their decision to keep me on. Whether it was not joining them or maintaining my distance when it came to personal conversations, no matter what, I won.

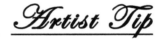

Artist Tip

- **Do your best work, get your money and go home.**

Masquerading
Victories

This chapter details expecting one thing (usually minor), only to have it evolve into something greater.

Success sometimes masquerades as hard work, and victories are occasionally hidden behind adversity. As you go through the motions, you'll discover a "small" door has morphed into a huge opportunity.

Such was the case when I was booked by a local businesswoman while still new to the industry. She loved her application, and referred me to the production company with whom she'd begun. The production company eventually secured the contract to produce commercials for a prestigious HBCU. Guess who was hired as the makeup artist?

One day while napping on the sofa in our family room with the television on, I heard a familiar script. My eyes popped open to recognize the face of the actress on the screen. It dawned on me - this was the commercial I'd done makeup for. I bolted straight up, in shock. Not only had I forgotten about filming it, I was elated to see my work on screen.

That HBCU commercial was the very first of many television ads I'd go on to do.

Once, I was referred by a former producer to do hair and makeup for a sports anchor. The test shoot was my trial; if hired, I'd work an hour a day, two days per week for two months. The pay was two hundred dollars an hour. I arrived at the station and when the talent arrived, her hair was completely different from the photos I'd seen during my research. When the producer interviewed me prior to the test shoot, I shared with him that hair wasn't my strong suit and he assured me the talent would come with her hair already done – my sole focus was makeup application.

The talent arrived with her hair partially wet and proceeded to pull extensions out of her purse. *Out of her purse!*

I was terrified, because I'd never touched a hair extension in my life. Without wanting to seem totally inept, I asked a few questions about her hair and how she preferred it to be styled. I had curlers, flat irons, hair spray and tools - all the necessary items needed to NOT style hair. But I digress…

She quickly explained how to clip in the extensions, before turning her attention to the script. I will be the first to tell you I jacked her hair up!!!! The front and sides were fabulous, but the extensions weren't properly secured in the back. I didn't clamp them in correctly; it seemed like they'd fall out at any moment. She was kind, smiling as she peered at herself in the mirror. I packed up and zipped out of there so fast, outracing the extensions before they hit the floor! It was AWFUL. I'm having a panic attack just thinking about it.

As I sat in the Uber on the way home, I emailed the producer to apologize about the hair. I reiterated I wasn't expecting to do hair - let alone extensions. He replied he thought everything went well, and he'd reach out once he confirmed with the talent.

...I never heard from him again.

I was devastated, partly because a former colleague had spoken so highly of me and I failed to deliver. Additionally, the finished application wasn't exemplary of my best work, and my name was on the line. Lastly, I was already looking forward to the salary I was promised. Four hundred dollars, two days a week, for a couple of months was a wonderful supplement to the other gigs I already had booked. The work for one talent would be so easy and the pay amazing. Thinking back on it - I was massacred!

Two weeks later, I received an email from another production company. I was referred by another former colleague, whom I'd worked with five years earlier. They were filming a pilot for two months. The rate was *five times* the rate of the gig I didn't get. I ended up getting selected and the show was extended for **FIVE** months.

You do the math...

Freelancing can be a balancing act. Sometimes, we must seriously consider whether the gig is worth our time to undertake. Because we're self-employed, we front our own expenses before seeing a dime of the money from the gig. The standard pay term is thirty days, so we might have to pay our own travel and lodging fees in advance, unless otherwise negotiated. To that end, we must assess whether it's even beneficial to accept a gig. Personally, I strive not to decline any money if I can help it; however, on occasion I've concluded all money isn't good money.

There are other times when the money isn't the greatest, but the gig has the potential to lead to other opportunities, or is a great addition to a résumé. Such was the case after relocating to New York, I received a request from a producer on the west coast, who would be in New York producing a commercial. After corresponding via email, I discovered the gig would be in the Hamptons. At the time, our home was just outside Jersey; since I don't like to drive very much, I strongly considered declining the gig. Filming happened to be on a Sunday, so my husband volunteered to drive me.

Have I told you guys how awesome he is?

Considering the three-hour drive to get there (one way), the pay wasn't that great; however, I had nothing booked for the day, and I was inspired by the deck. I hadn't done anything like this project since relocating, so it would be a nice addition to my portfolio. Traffic was horrendous, especially for a Sunday. The drive ended up being close to four hours thank goodness! I'm a fanatic about leaving extremely early to arrive at gigs on time.

Artist Tip

- **Good time management serves one well. Even if the project is delayed, I never want it to be delayed because of me. I've released several assistants due to their tardiness. My motto is:** *If you're on time, you're late.*

The shoot was slated for eight hours, so my hubby researched the area and decided to see a movie while we filmed. He dropped me off to a warm welcome from the rest of the crew. The talent was stunning and very pleasant as we discussed her makeup preferences. The atmosphere quickly dissolved my anxiety; filming was a blast! The next day, I received an email from the producer thanking me for my services…and offered me extra pay for the shoot. What a pleasant surprise!

Several months later, I received a call from another production company. They were producing a commercial to be aired during - wait for it…the Macy's Annual Thanksgiving Day Parade! I had worked with the talent on the commercial shoot in the Hamptons and she requested *me* as her makeup artist. To date, I've been her makeup artist for several commercials, all because of that initial project. Thank you, Taniya!

Was it a hassle to drive all the way out to the Hamptons in hella traffic? Yes.

Was it awkward meeting a new crew and performing a task I hadn't done before? Yes.

Was it worth it? Absolutely, YES!

Artist Tip

- **You may not immediately see the benefit, but trust me - it will manifest. Until it does, keep doing what you love, savor the moments, learn the lessons and perfect your craft. Enjoy the journey; you never know where it may lead.**

Mayvis Payne

There was another time when I arrived on set, and the PC seemed a bit aloof, and DP less than friendly. Throughout the day, I didn't have much interaction with the executives, and being this was my first time working with the team, I wasn't familiar with the talent or crew.

I noticed a particular gentleman tailing us as we filmed in the streets of New York City, however he was unassuming and seemed like an extra set of hands. The shoot carried on into the night; as we filmed the last scene, he stood by watching us take selfies. The all-male talent asked if they could take photos with me and I obliged. *I mean, it would be rude to deny eye candy, right?*

As we were wrapping, he approached me, said I did great work, and that he'd love to book me for many of their upcoming projects.

Sidebar: The afternoon of that shoot, I received an email from one of the producers, mentioning a colleague referred me to work on a multi-day shoot she was producing. The colleague she mentioned didn't sound familiar to me. I later discovered he was the same man who was speaking to me. He'd been admiring my work all day, and had sent emails to his colleagues.

This man wasn't a hired hand after all - he was the owner of the production company! Currently, I'm still on their roster of contractors, and for the past three years, I have traveled with them and worked on some of the greatest projects. In addition to being their go-to makeup artist, I was recommended (and hired) to work with some of their fellow filmmakers and colleagues. Some have since left the company, but continue to book me for projects. I could not have predicted the outcome; however, my expectations were definitely exceeded. The residual effects are very much worth it.

Red Carpets, Scarlet Rugs

I've had the privilege of accompanying some of the brightest stars on the red carpet. (You know I just had to take a selfie or two).

One of the most memorable carpet experiences came when I was hired to groom the handsome and debonair, Mack Wilds. He was just as cool as his television persona as I groomed him in his hotel suite. When we arrived at the carpet, security was weeding out "unnecessary" people to make room for the many celebrity guests. As I braced myself to be excused, I observed the lead guard informing various glam squads they had to leave. When he approached me, he whispered, "You must be someone special, because I was told that you have to remain put." I smiled and said thank you, marveling how divine favor had shown up once again!

Mack loved the way I groomed him, and the extra care I extended to ensure he was perfect for the red carpet. I mean, cameras were always snapping - he had to be picture perfect. As I was doting on him, he said, "I like you, Mom." To think I used to watch him on *The Wire* and now, I was styling him for the red carpet. I still call him my son, and I'm forever grateful for him granting me permission to include him in my book. I was smiling ear to ear, when he texted back, "Do it, Ma!"

Love me some him!

Another time while on the sidelines of the carpet, I heard my name when a celebrity was being interviewed. The host asked what or whom inspired him and he said "People like Mayvis Payne, who…. (I blacked out and didn't hear anything else after my name). Did I hear him correctly? He was looking directly at me when he said it, but I must've been dreaming.

He knew a bit of my story, and has always complimented me upon rising through the ranks. I mean, he was a huge star! I wanted to burst into tears when he said I was an inspiration to him.

Who? Little ol' me?

Once, I was surprised to receive a message from a television executive whom I hadn't seen in several years. She and I didn't have much interaction, but I admired her from afar. She wrote a magazine article and asked if she could include me as a celebrity artist. Of course, I was ecstatic, but I had no idea of the magnitude until she sent me a copy of the magazine. Not only was an extremely popular recording artist on the cover, but inside, my photo and introduction was directly beside a

HUGE celebrity artist. It was hilarious when a colleague called, asking if I knew I was featured alongside *him*. "I know," I casually replied...but, inside I was screaming.

This brings me to a conversation I once overheard. Two people were discussing the rate of a celebrity makeup artist and the star treatment she was receiving. Suddenly, one of them uttered a statement that pierced me – "She's *just* a makeup artist." His tone, the audacity in his inflection, the way he spewed it, gave me pause. But several years later, I began marketing myself as a celebrity makeup artist - to the disdain of some of my peers, and because of encouragement from others. Some thought I hadn't earned that title, since I'm not tied to a particular celebrity or traveling the globe with *A-listers*.

To be clear, although I am a *celebrity* artist, I'm a makeup artist first and foremost.

Period!

Though the celebrity title is true, it's not necessary. When you know who you are, titles don't matter. My title opened doors, but my work ethic has kept me inside. I was once told I couldn't simultaneously be a celebrity artist and work retail, but I've never fared well with people saying what I could not accomplish. If I wanted, I could very well return to retail beauty today, because I left in good standing with every brand I've ever worked with. And upon returning, I know how to lay my title aside, roll up my sleeves and do the work. I'm not a celebrity artist there...I'm an employee.

But again, when you know who you are...

Red carpet experiences are great, but small rug experiences keep you grounded.

In fact, the rugs have always been far greater.

Artist Tip

- **Don't get caught up in titles or how many celebrities you can work with. Offer the star treatment to everyone and watch doors fly open.**

A few years ago, I was encouraged to reinvent myself, particularly my cosmetic brand - It's all about branding. Under my brand, I have a collection of lip glosses, lipsticks and lip stains. *Insert shameless plug here: www.getloxed.com.*

I prefer to liken my experience in this industry to the variety of lip products:

Lip Glosses: These are the things you either don't address or give any lingering thought. Simply gloss over it. Don't allow it to affect the way you conduct yourself or your business. These are events you chalk up to, "It's not a big deal, it's not that serious, and doesn't deserve anymore of my energy."

A lip gloss moment for me was when a talent was upset because I couldn't make her look like the picture of Kim Kardashian she had shown me. Mind you, her facial shape, eyelids and bone structure were drastically different. She was at least twenty-five years older than Kim; even her ethnicity was different. Honey, I couldn't have made her look like Kim, even with a magic wand! She bad-mouthed me to her assistant, but I was unbothered.

Lip gloss applied.

Then, there are other experiences which leave you wounded.

These are the **Lip Stains**: they hurt, are uncomfortable, and may affect how you move forward or prohibit you from doing so. You can't gloss these over; the pain or disappointment is a constant reminder of what happened. You must acknowledge it and let it take its course. Only then can healing begin; only then can you proceed...but do so with caution.

You can wipe off a lip stain, but if you don't remove it properly, the residue remains. If you allow these occasions to deeply affect you, the damage remains long after the situation has ended. These are the experiences which can morph into teaching moments; learn something from it and allow it to work to your advantage. I've had more lip stain moments than I can recall. It would take at least three more chapters, and who has that amount of time?

My most memorable lip stain experiences have resulted from relationships I've formed. Those are the hardest, because some relationships I thought would last forever, but for whatever reason ended. Whether it was a celebrity, talent or colleague, I must conclude they served their purpose and their season in my life is over.

Remember seasons change.

Did it hurt? Heck yeah (still)

Was it fair? Nope.

What are you going to do about it? Move on.

This one is poignant, because in my experience, it's often been at the hands of those whom I've helped along the way. Some took my assistance, then turned their back on me; there were others I helped get recognized, and their career took off before mine. Or, worse yet - I bent over backwards helping them achieve their goals... in return, they acted as if they never knew me. Or when I needed their help, they said no. That still stings. But it won't always, it's only a stain.

Mayvis Payne

One time, I invited someone I helped get her foot in the door for lunch. We hadn't seen each other in about a year or so. She kept talking about how she was working with another artist, and how he'd been calling her to assist on gigs. My career wasn't what it became and I think she considered him to be her claim to fame. Now this was the same guy whom she knew was backstabbing and bad-mouthing me just a few years earlier. It wasn't just the fact that she was working with him, it was the *WAY* she idolized him and was enamored about working with him, even though she knew firsthand the things he did to me. Heck, she was with me when I first discovered it! In the long run, I believe she thought his opportunities would somehow become hers, so she'd better get on his good side (translation: kiss his butt to get ahead).

Sidebar: I wonder whatever happened to them - I never hear anything about either of them anymore.

Something about our conversation that day made me super uneasy; however, it was very enlightening. I treated her to lunch, and it was money well spent, knowing it would be our final meal together.

Many years later, I received a request from her asking if she could join me at one of my star-studded events. I'm not bitter, but I'm no fool. What! You mean, he can't get you on the guest list? Oh, I forgot; he wasn't invited.

Invitation declined.

There are many more stains I've been dealt, and I'm certain there will be more. Instances such as these have taught me to be more cautious in allowing people into my professional circle. It has also resulted in me being much more selective in what I share and disclose. Even when it comes to penning this book - very few were aware of it.

If there's one thing this industry has taught me throughout the years, it is to move in silence. There is always a method to my madness; I have become quite strategic about information sharing.

Although there are many instances of negative energy, I choose to dwell on the positive things which propel me to a greater version of myself.

These are the **Lipstick** experiences: the events and situations which leave an indelible impression. Just like actual lipstick, these occurrences can be altered to color your life as needed. The setting might change, but the lesson forever remains.

Most of my lipstick moments stem from private conversations or encounters I've had, either with a celebrity client or a personal on-set encounter. I don't dare disclose them, but they're the ones I'll cherish forever. If there's a theme defining lipstick moments, it is that celebrities are people, just like you and me. Prior to working with them, I admit I was super judgmental if I heard of someone's negative encounter with a star; however, whether behind the scenes or up close, I must also admit my perspective has changed. Although I've experienced the negativity firsthand, I now try to put myself in their shoes. Most of us have no idea of the pressures that celebrity status brings.

One time, I was among a group of people who were discussing a particular celebrity as if they knew her personally. They had no idea that I worked with celebrity clientele, let alone I'd worked with this particular one on several occasions. They were ripping her apart! Typically, I would've remained silent, but I considered this a teachable (lipstick) moment.

As each one offered their biting critique of her, I recalled a private conversation she and I had years earlier. When there was a pause in the conversation, I very calmly and pointedly offered this advice – "Most of us are a millisecond away from becoming someone even we wouldn't recognize. Given the perfect environment and opportunity, we might find ourselves doing something we swore we would never do."

Conversation was immediately over. Drop the mic. Case closed!

The awkward silence and stoic expressions assured me that my words had hit their mark. I didn't disclose I'd worked with her, nor the details of our conversation; I simply offered another perspective. If I hadn't had a personal encounter with her, I may not have been able to silence the discourse. Sometimes, the only thing needed is for someone to step up and silence the noise.

Another time, a relative of mine discovered I had the personal phone number of a celebrity client. He asked why I hadn't told him I had the number when he was such a huge fan. Having a celebrity's contact information is no reason to brag, disrespect their privacy or usurp authority. Their respect is a privilege; I would be wise to preserve their trust and privacy. As stylists, we are privy to some of their most vulnerable moments, and it would behoove us to rise above the status quo.

That brings me to the celebrity client who kept dozing off during her makeover, because she was exhausted from travel and had just come in from a flight. Instead of compromising her integrity by waking her up, I held her head up with one hand, and groomed her with the other. When she woke up, she was appreciative and thanked me for allowing her to sleep. Although it was a bit unconventional and slightly inconvenient, I kept her comfortable. That's the end goal.

Another time, a client I was grooming in a crowded makeup studio had a medical crisis. Not only was the room full of handlers, crew, and other celebrities, it was also where photographers were constantly snapping pictures and taking videos. As I noticed her slipping into unconsciousness, I quickly turned her chair away from public view and discreetly motioned for one of the producers, who motioned for another person, who quietly began praying, as we garnered medical attention.

When she was finally coherent, the client couldn't stop thanking us - specifically for protecting her. In a social media driven world, the situation could've ended up viral before we knew it; she understood our fast-acting saved her from embarrassment had everyone noticed the event. Later, she shared her condition with me; I prayed for her in that area, as well as watched out for her when working together.

Another time, my husband accompanied me to an after party chocked full of celebrities. One of the celebrities I groomed introduced himself to my husband, and asked if I were his wife. When my husband said yes, the celebrity told him I was a riot as he shook his hand and congratulated him. (I'm assuming that was a good thing). An hour later, one of my hubby's favorite artists came over and asked if we'd watch her drink while she danced. Of all the people in the room, she asked us. I had never styled her before, but apparently, she felt comfortable enough to approach us. Besides, the way my hubby practically hollered "Yes," with a giant grin plastered on his face, there's no way I would've refused. You couldn't tell him anything after that; he was a fan before – now he's a fanatic! He has convinced himself that she had the hots for him.

Oh well, let him have his dream...but, you're stuck with me, baby!

Contrary to popular belief, a lot of my most-celebrated memories involve regular people, or famous clients who have become dear friends. For instance, one of my favorite red carpet moments didn't happen on the carpet. It was because of a text I received from one of London's top news anchors and current client, Emily Maitlis. I was delighted when I awakened to read, "Mayvis! I wrote a book and you're in it!" Her text rang with as much excitement as I had while reading it.

For someone of her status to even consider me is a distinct honor. And to include me in the story of the James Comey interview? Beyond epic!

Oddly enough, I felt that same euphoria when one of my *regular* clients included me in her book - although Miss LaWan is anything but regular!

Another time, I got the red-carpet treatment when I traveled (at my own expense) to surprise a former celebrity client for her birthday. When I checked into the hotel, I was upgraded to the Presidential Suite, due to my relationship with one of the artists. While in town, I ended up booking a video/photo shoot with another artist, and was pleasantly surprised to discover that all my meals had been comped when I returned to the hotel. That artist and I are very good friends; we have vacationed together, we know each other's families and we share a special bond.

Another time while checking into a hotel for a weekend

celebrity event, the front-desk agent excused herself for a moment. When she returned, she placed an 8x10 photo frame on the check-in counter, and told me that she was upgrading me to the penthouse suite.

As I stood in line, I heard whispers and turned to see people in line behind me, pointing and waving. I had never been to this area before; of course, they weren't waving at me. I shrugged it off, until I received my room key and stepped to the side to gather my things. It was then that I saw it: the frame displayed my picture with the caption, **Welcome Celebrity Makeup Artist, Mayvis Payne**.

I was floored! I'd never met this woman before, and she never said a word; she just instantly made my day. Not only did I receive numerous requests for makeovers during my stay, but when I checked out a couple of days later, someone had paid my hotel bill.

These are only a fraction of the Lipstick Moments I hold dear, to remain in my heart forever. I hope to keep sentiments like these in the forefront of my mind, to be mindful of my behavior. As one of my friends put it: "What you build with your gift, you can destroy with your character."

Artist Tip

- **Read that again.**

Whether on the red carpet or a red rug, remain consistent and integral. Your character is on display at all times and you'd be surprised who notices.

Idol Eyes

O ne of my favorite cosmetic brands used to have an eye shadow called *Idol Eyes*. It was shiny and chocked full of glitter, which is what attracted me to it. I was hooked from the moment I saw it, although the background of the shadow kind of faded and paled in comparison to the brightness of the glitter. I discovered that without the security of the color underneath, the glitter had no longevity. In other words - it quickly fell off and disappeared. Without the proper foundation, it lacked staying power.

This chapter is dedicated to those who support the stars, so they can shine. These are the ones who are rarely acknowledged; however, they are the foundation of the industry. Of course, we don't idolize them- we only want to get a glimpse of celebrities, but these are the ones who help the stars to succeed.

Mayvis Payne

We are the ones behind the scenes, instrumental in the success of the star vehicle. In a well-oiled machine, we are the oil. *We got the juice!*

Today, I salute each producer, production coordinator, stagehand, PA, hairstylist, makeup artist, assistant, wardrobe stylist, gaffer, grip, photographer, AC, DP, craft services personnel, janitor, driver, gatekeeper, spouse, family member, culinary director, etc.

We don't always receive our just reward, and very few of us enjoy the honor of seeing our name as an award recipient; however, our work should be celebrated. I endeavor to always celebrate award winners, whether I know them or not. Additionally, I'm *that* person who remains seated in the theater, just to read the credits at the end of the film. Not to see who the characters are, but to read the names of the makeup artists and hairstylists. Society has encouraged competition, but I choose to believe there's room for all of us. To that end, I celebrate the accomplishments of others.

There are makeup artists whose products I've purchased, yet they have never supported my endeavors, purchased my products, nor even acknowledged me - I know they see me! Perhaps they don't consider me to be on their level, but I don't gain value from their validation, or lack thereof. Had I entertained the opinion of naysayers, I would never have had a career in the industry, and you wouldn't be reading my story.

Who would've known when I purchased my first make up book, I'd be mentioned in one, let alone write one? One day, while conducting a Google search, I saw a mention of my name. But it wasn't simply a mention, it was with whom my name was included - the industry greats! I'll never forget it, as long as I live.

Shout out to my makeup daughter, Vanessa, whom I affectionately called VBA.

And, speaking of my daughter, I had to laugh when my biological daughter called me one day and squealed, "Mommmmm," (yes, she drew it out in an elongated syllable, as only she can), did you know that you're Google-able?" She was so excited. I did know, but hadn't given it much thought. I was simply stacking the coins and adding to my résumé; doing what I love. It's not the attention of celebrities I most admire; it's the respect of my peers, friends, and family members. VBA, Meghan, Shannyn, Andrea, Kayla, and Bella (among others) have assisted me on some of my greatest projects and I'm forever grateful to them. They have helped me achieve some of my biggest goals, and have assisted in bringing my vision to fruition.

Some of the industry's best producers have entrusted my services to their projects and I am indebted to them forever: Wendy, Donna, Ian, Lynn, Torrence, Eric, Rashonda, Stephanie, Crystal, Lindsay, Adam, Mike, Chris, Darren, Jamie, Krista, Gideon, Sean, Brian, John, Victoria, Julia, Joe, Christian, Lance and many others. (My memory is sketchy in my older age, so I should probably stop naming names).

If I've worked on any of your projects, let me say *THANK YOU*. My career could not have been what it is, had it not been for your belief in me. Some have been introduced as clients, but remained as friends. Some have become acquaintances or even enemies; however, their contribution to my success should not be ignored. It takes both water and dirt to make flowers grow.

Mayvis Payne

A huge shout out to fellow makeup artists, who entrusted me with their clients. Whether you felt sorry for me (ha-ha), or genuinely wanted me to succeed, I appreciate the referrals and the residuals.

...except the MUA who wanted me to do a ten-hour photo shoot with a celebrity artist and band for two hundred dollars.

After deducting tolls, gas and parking, I would have netted about forty-eight dollars. No ma'am - you are not included in this gracious thank you note, LOL!

But seriously, even the rejections, closed doors and being ignored, deserve a shout out. If not for those, I probably would not completely appreciate the successes I've enjoyed. A special shout out to my friends for allowing me to practice on their faces. Also, friends who shared my contact information, posted on their pages or simply supported by word of mouth.

I appreciate you.

To the fellow makeup artists whom I have worked alongside on countless sets without competing with me. Oh yeah, a special thank you to that one glam team out west, who didn't want me to be in the same makeup room with them. Because of you, I had to work in another corridor, which happened to house the biggest celebrities of the show.

What an awesome honor to add them to my résumé!

It was especially rewarding to discover some of them left your chairs to have me groom them instead.

Oh, the irony.

Thank you to the makeup department heads who took a chance bringing me in, even though I was new to the game. Likewise, a shout out to those who didn't hire me for the same reason. I developed a thick skin, which everyone needs in this industry.

I'd like to thank the aspiring makeup artists who have reached out to me over the years, either to glean from me or to seek my advice. Consequently, I've offered each one the same advice – Research, research, research. Some have been upset by my response; however, although I am an advocate for helping - I also recognize the value in researching for yourself. Trust me, it's likely the best free advice you will ever receive.

And please, don't allow anyone to crush your dreams. Whatever you do, don't give up and remember to trust the process.

One year, I was in a show's audience laughing at the host's jokes. Two years later, I was his personal makeup artist for the very same show. Do what you must, until you can do what you want. During one of my lean times, I got a job as an early morning stock clerk to assist my hubby with bills. Two years later, he rewarded me by agreeing to uproot our family to New York, so I could live my dream. Don't be so haughty that you turn down other jobs because they're not what you want to do. It's a means to an end. Heck, I still return to freelancing from time to time, if I need to supplement my income or if I'm working towards a personal goal.

I began my career as a makeup artist in 2004. Four years earlier, I was a single mother and homeless! Eight years later, I moved to New York to advance my career.

When one of my colleagues discovered I was relocating, he asked why I would move to an area so saturated with makeup artists. He saw it as major competition; I viewed it as a major opportunity. We are not the same; perspective is paramount.

This industry can bite, but when you know who you are and

what you're called to do, you can accomplish anything.

And how could I ever forget those who have attended my seminars, makeup classes and purchased my video tutorials. I'm grateful you have entrusted me to teach you. There are so many experts in this industry, and I appreciate you for allowing me the opportunity to share my knowledge.

The directors and producers who put in long hours to present pilots are my heroes as well. Especially those whose projects never see the light of day. I've worked on some of those projects, and can imagine how devastating it is when your vision is rejected. I'm nonetheless inspired by them, because they keep writing, presenting, pursuing, and dreaming.

To my private clients - whether you hired me for your wedding, daughter's prom or graduation, black-tie event, conference or seminar…I appreciate you. You are the ones who keep me grounded, and the ones who refer me to friends, coworkers and family members.

To the mother of the groom who requested that I apply a shiny, black lipstick for her son's wedding. Sorry; not sorry!

She was so upset with me; hope she got over it.

A ton of gratitude to the makeup artists who paved the way for those of us who desire to work in this industry. Even before the term *celebrity makeup artist* became a thing, it was your art and wisdom we sought to emulate. A special thanks to those of you who took the time to impart into my life; there are some whom I've admired from afar, others up close and personal. Whatever your contribution, I appreciate you - particularly your perseverance and willingness to adapt within this ever-evolving craft.

I would be remiss if I failed to mention Trish. After sitting in my chair, she decided to interview me on her radio show, not once, but several times. She follows my journey and offers me a platform to share upcoming appearances and new product launches. I've never asked for a spot, she features me on her own, and I appreciate her for that.

To my immediate and extended family: Thank you.

It's been said those most familiar with you don't support you; however, that's not my testimony. My cousins, aunts, uncles, and friends have blessed my life and supported my business ventures...tremendously!

Lastly, but most importantly, I thank my dear husband, Michael R. Payne. It's because of your insistence that I pursued becoming a makeup artist in the first place. Your unwavering love and support has single-handedly undergirded (i.e., financed) my career.

Thank you for doubling as my driver, also. The countless 4:00 a.m. commutes, 1:00 a.m. pick-up times, the shuffling of your work schedule to ensure I had safe transportation, the holding down of the fort (mortgage, bills, groceries and luxuries) during the lean times, when I had no money coming in, are greatly appreciated. I'm not sure if you fully saw the vision, but if you didn't, you never let me know it.

We did it, baby! I couldn't have done it without you, nor would I want to. Of all my many accomplishments, marrying you tops the list! Who would've known when you saw me walking down the hall in a neck and back brace, that we'd be where we are?

Thank you for being my biggest cheerleader.

I may be faintly admired by some, but I'm completely loved by ONE.

Exit Stage Left

We have possibly closed out one of the most challenging years in history. Actually - THE WORST. 2020 was nobody's punk. It dealt the kind of one-two punch that takes your breath away. It was the kind of slap to the face that stung like reaching the top step of the subway station on a cold, windy day.

Yeah, that kind…

The second week of March 2020, my client/job market and wages dried up, my husband had a heart attack, and our daughter was hospitalized with the virus and pneumonia. Our prospects seemed grim, to put it mildly.

Although extremely challenging *for* me, it was equally rewarding *to* me. Just look: You are holding in your hands the fruit of my labor!

Mayvis Payne

What else did I have to do? What excuse could I use?

New York City is closed. I, as well as many others have lost our income due to the Coronavirus pandemic. No early morning treks to the train, late evening wrap times, or shuffling people out of the way on busy sidewalks. (Maybe I'm the only one who does that).

No meeting up with my friends for a late-night bite to eat, no blaring of the yellow taxi horns, or squinting to peer at the license plate of the Uber driver. Production has ceased, Broadway is silenced, restaurants are shuttered, hopes are dashed, and dreams are deferred. Or, are they?

Perhaps, it is the perfect time to dust off that goal that you've been putting off...I did.

I miss being in the city. I hope its absence has brought about a great appreciation of the arts, which seemed to have been lost prior to the pandemic. Though not necessarily essential workers (whom I have mad respect for), artists should be celebrated and encouraged.

My daughter was bragging about how as a single mother, I encouraged my kids' involvement in extracurricular activities, sports and art. She must've forgotten how elated I was when my son's drums got a hole in them and I could finally throw them out.

Or the time he was spanked for drawing all over her brand-new stereo and the walls with bright, colorful crayons. *Creativity stifled.*

Maybe I will get my Oscar after all...is there a *Bad Parent* category?

Though my revenue has waned, I have a different perspective. The unwelcomed recess has afforded me the

124

awesome opportunity of penning my story.

But why this story you may ask?

First, I must let you in on a secret. This book has been years in the making. I knew I had a story to tell (and people kept reminding me), but I kept putting it on the back burner.

Besides, I would tell myself, who would buy my book? What would more successful, more seasoned artists think? Who am I that people would even want to hear what I have to say? Would my clients approve? What if I fail?

All these questions and more were squashed as soon as I committed to writing. It's destiny. I *had* to write it. If not for you, for me. Therapy wasn't the intent, but peace comes when you stop kicking against the pricks and embrace your calling.

I teach makeup because when I started, no one was willing to teach me about the industry. Sadly, we've created a culture that would prefer to foster competition than camaraderie. We've become miserly, covetous and fearful of being second best. If I must become second best, I will be the greatest at it, because it would be MY best!

I think that's what's lost on most of us. We've been duped into thinking if we teach someone anything new, they'll be better than we are at it. But isn't that the goal? To leave someone better than we found them? It should be.

I hope that every assistant I've had, go on to do greater exploits and achieve greater success than I've enjoyed.

I was once told, "You give too much information away when you teach."

My response? "If I gave someone my entire kit, they might do the job better than me, but they could never *be* me."

The doors meant to open for me will open, and I'll kindly

walk right through them. That's a golden nugget I'd love to cement in someone's psyche. There will always be someone who does what you do, better. There's a young teenager out there somewhere, who can paint you right out of a job. But so be it; just do *you*!

There are some seasoned artists who say I'm irrelevant because I don't have enough movie credits, haven't worked with the right A-listers, or haven't accomplished what they have, but I'm comfortable in my own skin. Traffic on the freeway doesn't bother me, if I'm focused on my own lane. Besides, my resume isn't too shabby, either!

If there's a central theme 2020 has taught us, I hope it is this: *Get over ourselves*. From racial inequality, police brutality, escalated unemployment, unfathomable death toll and political chaos, we have loads of work to do. Speaking of race, I have experienced my share of racial bias in this industry, but I refuse to allow those instances to stop me. To the contrary, it made me more determined. I've witnessed the disdain, sneers, whispers and dirty looks. I've had my services declined because of my skin color.

I recall an executive pulling me aside, away from an all-white crew, asking if I was sure I could do *white makeup*. I knew what she was alluding to, but I responded in a manner deemed professionally sarcastic.

"Do you mean like mimes?" I asked. *Clearly more sarcastically than professional.*

Once, while freelancing for a luxury brand in an exclusive boutique, a mother didn't want me to apply hers, nor her daughters' makeup because - in her words, "Well, she's black." I glanced at the mirror in feigned horror and gasped, "I am!?!?"

126

Refusing to entertain her foolishness, the manager had a quick word with the rude woman, then escorted one of the girls to my chair. After completing the first daughter's makeup, the mother and her other daughter insisted I do theirs. Afterwards, they requested my contact information and purchased everything I suggested. By the way - the manager advised me that after reprimanding the mother, she assured her I was the most experienced and talented artist in the room.

Another time, a young lady arrived for her appointment, and when the manager introduced me as her artist, she requested a white girl do her makeup (different brand, different boutique...same story). The manager told her none were available; I saw her body tense as I selected the products for her makeover.

"You're going to put *that* color on my eyes?" She asked through clenched teeth with a roll of the eyes.

"Yep," I replied cheerfully. I endured the silent treatment and stiff neck, finished her makeover, and kindly handed her a mirror to critique my work.

She tipped me fifty dollars, asked for my contact information and became one of my private clients. Later, she confided that the people at the event I dolled her up for couldn't stop raving about her makeup...particularly *that* eyeshadow.

My point?

When you get down to it, we're all the same. Flawed, yet special in ways which might not be immediately seen. Sometimes, it takes someone else to quiet the noise and offer another perspective. I've said this earlier, but it bears repeating.

I appreciate the manager for sticking to her guns and not allowing the customer to control the narrative.

But why should skin even matter? Why does someone's

Mayvis Payne

social status have to enter the equation?

It should be of no importance that your clients are more famous or richer than mine. We all have goals, let's work together to achieve them.

In other words, can we just do the work, love and respect each other and move forward?

Please and thank you.

Throughout 2020, we've endured so much racial tension, it's sickening. I'm happy for the enlightening, which has resulted in support for racial equality. **Black Lives Matter!**

This memoir is a personal goal of mine. I've accomplished a feat I didn't think possible. "She won't ever amount to anything," a family member once said of me. "Probably won't do anything except have a bunch of babies."

Decades later, I have two children, and can run down my list of accomplishments; thank you very much. I showed her!

Remember, I was never very fond of others writing my story. I am told that she brags about me behind my back...never to me personally, but oh well; she got the memo!

You might not like my story. You may even disagree with it, or the way I've chosen to express it. You might think it's too much, not enough, or too soon, but it's my story, told through my lens, the way I want. It is the first week of a new year and my first goal has been completed.

Take that, 2020!

We have no idea where 2021 is headed, but I'm not resting on my laurels while I wait. There are other opportunities waiting to be discovered, uncovered and explored. I hope by sharing my story, you'll be inspired to tell your own. I hope someone who reads this book can avoid the pitfalls and disappointments

I've encountered. Even if you experience less-than-ideal circumstances, I hope this book serves as a blueprint on how to better handle them. *Feel free to learn from my mistakes; I don't need the credit.*

It's my aim to inform and inspire, enlighten and encourage, and to likewise urge someone to pursue and persevere. That sounded like a three-point Sunday sermon, but I want you to know that dreams DO come true. But make sure it's your dream, and not merely a wish to be like anyone else.

Lastly, I pray we all would be kinder to one another, especially those who are walking a different path than ours. I'm in the business of external beauty, but a beautiful soul should always shine through. Trust me, I've seen some of the most beautifully made-up faces, with garbage receptacles for souls.

Once, I was asked what is the one thing I would say to celebrities, that I wish they all knew.

It is this:

Forget the egos and royal personas. Never be too famous to be nice. I get it – you're tired, having a horrible day, and just want to be left alone. But consider that a simple, small and kind gesture could brighten a fan's day. You are in the spotlight. If you must show up, put your best face forward. Don't just show up; SHINE!

The same advice could be offered to all of us, especially those of us in the entertainment field. It doesn't matter who you are, what your role is or the success you've obtained. Everyone deserves kindness; be the light. But what do I know?

I'm *just* a makeup artist.

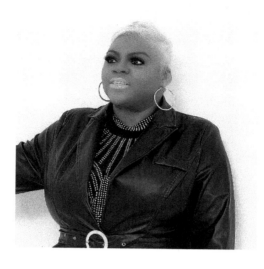

About The Author

Mayvis Payne is a New York-based makeup artist with more than fifteen years of experience in film/television, digital, bridal, runway and retail beauty. Although known as a Celebrity Makeup Artist, her passion is making the *everyday* client beautiful. She's often heard saying, "Everybody's a star in my chair!"

Mayvis has worked with celebrities such as T.I., Common, the late Dr. Maya Angelou, Piers Morgan, James Comey, Tatyana Ali, Cissy Houston and countless others. Mayvis has worked behind the scenes on such shows as *Black Girls Rock, BET Honors, Being Mary Jane Reunion, Celebration of Gospel, My Grandmother's Ravioli, RuPaul's Drag Race Red Carpet, 106 & Party*, to name a few.

Her television credits include: *A&E, Bloomberg Television,*

Mayvis Payne

BBC News, Cooking Channel, ESPN, Food Network, Fuse, Lifetime, NatGeo, NBC, News12NJ, SuperBowl Gospel, TV Land, TVOne, WE TV and countless others.

For bio, complete client list and bookings, you may visit www.mayvispayne.com.

Acknowledgements:

My Lord and Savior, Jesus Christ for everything
Michael R. Payne
Mo Rocca
Gideon Evans
Karen Gale Tuttle
T. Pain
John McPherson (BBC News)
Piers Morgan
Emily Maitlis (BBC)
Lindsey Christian (Director, Producer, Co-Writer)
Tristan Mack Wilds
Samantha Seneviratne
Krista Linney (Maiden Creative)
C. Williams
Torrence Glenn
Eric Rhett (Production Manager, Citizen Jones)
Taniya Nayak
Stephanie Madison
Trish Standley
Quincy Brownlee Adesokan
Charron Monaye
Don Panama
Pen Legacy Team